A CLINICIAN'S GUIDE TO PALLIATIVE CARE

To :

Dr. Richard Payne —
Leader in American
Pain medicine, friend and
Colleague —
Jerry Kmenent

April 29, 2004

A CLINICIAN'S GUIDE TO PALLIATIVE CARE

George J. Taylor, MD
Professor of Medicine
Division of Cardiology
Department of Medicine
Medical University of South Carolina
Charleston, South Carolina

Jerome E. Kurent, MD, MPH
Associate Professor of Medicine, Neurology, and Psychiatry
Division of General Internal Medicine/Geriatrics
Department of Medicine
Medical University of South Carolina
Charleston, South Carolina

Blackwell
Publishing

© 2003 by Blackwell Science
a Blackwell Publishing company

Blackwell Publishing, Inc.,
350 Main Street, Malden, Massachusetts 02148-5018, USA
Blackwell Publishing Ltd, 9600 Garsington Road, Oxford OX4 2DQ, UK
Blackwell Science Asia Pty Ltd,
550 Swanston Street, Carlton South, Victoria 3053, Australia
Blackwell Verlag GmbH, Kurfürstendamm 57, 10707 Berlin, Germany

02 03 04 05 5 4 3 2 1

ISBN: 0-632-04642-2

Library of Congress Cataloging-in-Publication Data

A clinician's guide to palliative care / [edited by] George J. Taylor,
Jerome E. Kurent.
    p. ; cm.
Includes bibliographical references and index.
    ISBN 0-632-04642-2 (pbk.)
    1. Palliative treatment.   2. Terminal care.   3. Terminally ill.
    [DNLM: 1. Palliative Care.   2. Chronic Disease—therapy. WB 310
    C6415 2003]   I. Taylor, George Jesse.   II. Kurent, Jerome E.

R726.8 .C576 2003
616′.029—dc21
                                                        2002015312

A catalogue record for this title is available from the British Library

Acquisitions: Beverly Copland
Development: Amy Nuttbrock
Production: Jennifer Kowalewski
Cover design: Eve Siegel
Typesetter: SNP Best-set Typesetter Ltd., in Hong Kong
Printed and bound by Malloy Lithographing, Inc., in Ann Arbor, MI

For further information on Blackwell Publishing, visit our website:
www.medirect.com

Notice: The indications and dosages of all drugs in this book have been
recommended in the medical literature and conform to the practices of the
general community. The medications described do not necessarily have specific
approval by the Food and Drug Administration for use in the diseases and
dosages for which they are recommended. The package insert for each drug
should be consulted for use and dosage as approved by the FDA. Because
standards for usage change, it is advisable to keep abreast of revised
recommendations, particularly those concerning new drugs.

Dedication

To our parents, for their gifts of love and support

   Fannie Chance Taylor
   George J. Taylor III*
   Catherine Louise Reiners*
   Bernard M. Reiners*

and

   Anne D. Kurent*
   Edward A. Kurent, Sr.*
   Richard G. Warner*
   Barbara D. Warner

* Deceased

Contents

Foreword

The Institute of Medicine in 1997 issued its report, "Approaching Death," on the state of medical care for the dying in the United States and identified serious inadequacies in the current provision of care to dying persons and their families. The report singled out health care professionals' lack of knowledge and lack of training in palliative care as major barriers and called for the need to educate health care professionals with the essential attitudes, skills, and knowledge to care well for dying patients. Emphasizing the importance of integrating palliative care approaches into the continuum of care for all patients, the report called for the translation of existing palliative care principles and practice into the everyday care of the dying.

A Clinician's Guide to Palliative Care takes up this educational imperative and serves as a practical resource for primary care physicians describing appropriate, competent, humane end-of-life care. This text starts with the general outline of the approach to the care of a person with a life ending illness and uses specific disease management chapters to provide the practical symptom assessment and management strategies. From the management of the patient with end-stage renal disease to the care of the advanced cancer patient, the chapters focus on those common illnesses that cause the majority of deaths in the United States— heart disease, cancer, neurodegenerative diseases, major organ failure, and AIDS. The last two chapters focus on special populations, children and the elderly in nursing homes, detailing the important and relevant ethical and symptom management challenges for these vulnerable groups.

At the book's outset, the authors with years of clinical experience in caring for the seriously ill describe their perspectives on the goals of medicine: to prolong life, to improve the quality of life, and to assure a good death. The uniqueness of this text is in the authors' accepting the health care professionals' responsibility to address patients' distress and to reduce their needless suffering. Communication skills are identified as critical to facilitate physicians' competency and comfort to initiate and sustain difficult physician, patient, and family conversations when defining the goals of care and acknowledging death as an inevitable outcome. Such "death talk," when sensitive and appropriate to the needs of the patient and family, can assure the patient that their autonomy will be respected, their dignity preserved, and their symptoms managed. Each disease specific chapter tries to model these conversations with the authors providing their personal perspectives on how they conduct such conversations.

By combining state of the art medical management with evidence-based symptom control approaches, this guide models the routinization of palliative care in primary care medicine. By modeling for clinicians how to walk the last mile with their patients with competency, sound judgment, and compassion, this guide serves to educate health care professionals to help their patients "negotiate life's final transition."

As Anatole Broyard, who was dying from cancer, poignantly observed, "the doctor has little to lose and everything to gain by letting the sick man into his heart. If he does, they can share as few others the wonder, terror, and exultation of being on the edge of being."

Kathleen M. Foley, MD
Attending Neurologist, Memorial Sloan Kettering Cancer Center
Professor of Neurology, Neuroscience & Clinical Pharmacology
Weill Medical College of Cornell University
Director, Project on Death in America

Preface

At some point in most person's lives, the goal of medical care becomes a good and peaceful death. Helping patients with this experience should be a rewarding aspect of practice. Yet, many doctors find it stressful. Our culture of scientific medicine places greatest emphasis on curing disease, and few of us have had specific training in the management of dying patients. On the contrary, "losing" a patient is perceived as a failure of medicine, and most physicians are reluctant to "give up."

A Clinician's Guide to Palliative Care emphasizes that an effective doctor does not give up, but rather shifts to a palliative model of care when cure is no longer possible. Its premise is that sound clinical judgment, good planning and communication, sensitivity, and compassion will allow you to do great good.

There is a brief discussion of general principles of palliation, and of ethical issues at end of life. This practical medical text also has chapters reviewing chronic illnesses in addition to cancer— congestive heart failure, liver disease, renal failure, coronary artery disease, AIDS, obstructive lung disease, and debilitating neurological diseases. We review the natural history of these conditions, addressing how to determine when a patient is end-stage, and when palliative care is preferable. We discuss drug and/or interventional therapies that prolong survival but that are also used for the control of symptoms. A separate chapter reviews the pharmacology of pain relief and symptom control. Two brief chapters address special issues in pediatric palliation and the frail elderly nursing home resident.

Throughout, we describe how we communicate and face tough decisions with patients and families. For instance, how might you tell an unsuspecting patient that the illness is fatal? What advance directive is needed, and is it fail-safe? What are the hospice admission criteria? Are there legal issues that influence decision-making? When making decisions what are the roles of the doctor, the family, and non-family caregivers?

We are indebted to the chapter contributors who drew on their extensive experience and unique expertise to make *A Clinician's*

Guide to Palliative Care a reality. We wrote *A Clinician's Guide to Palliative Care* for primary care practitioners, medical students, and house officers. It was written especially for those of you who are uncomfortable with aggressive treatment of patients with advanced disease when the chance of benefit is limited and treatment increases suffering. Our aim is to present the "big picture," and this is not an exhaustive review. As a general introduction, we hope that you read it through, roughly a three-evening project.

George J. Taylor, MD
Jerome E. Kurent, MD, MPH*

*Faculty Scholar, Project on Death in America, 2000–2002.
Dr. Kurent gratefully acknowledges the Open Society Institute for its generous support.

Contributors

Frank J. Brescia, MD, PACP
Attending Oncologist
Hollings Cancer Center
Professor of Medicine
Medical University of South Carolina
Charleston, South Carolina

Lewis M. Cohen, MD
Co-Director of Consultation Psychiatry
Baystate Medical Center
Springfield, Massachusetts
Associate Professor of Psychiatry
Tufts University School of Medicine
Medford, Massachusetts

John E. Heffner, MD
Executive Medical Director
Professor of Medicine
Medical University of South Carolina
Charleston, South Carolina

Jerome E. Kurent, MD, MPH
Associate Professor of Medicine, Neurology, and Psychiatry
Division of General Internal Medicine/Geriatrics
Department of Medicine
Medical University of South Carolina
Charleston, South Carolina

Harlee S. Kutzen, MN, ACRN
HIV Palliative Care Nurse Specialist
Louisiana State University Health Sciences Center
Palliative Care Principal Investigator
HIV Division of Medicine
Louisiana State University
New Orleans, Louisiana

Kristi L. Lenz, PharmD
Oncology Clinical Pharmacist
Medical University Hospital
Associate Professor of Pharmacy
Medical University of South Carolina
Charleston, South Carolina

David M. Poppel, MD
Nephrologist
Western New England Renal & Transplant Association
Associate Clinical Professor of Medicine
Tufts Medical School (Baystate Medical Center)
Springfield, Massachusetts

Dale Anne Singer, MD
Department of Hematology/Oncology
Phoenix Children's Hospital
Phoenix, Arizona

George J. Taylor, MD
Professor of Medicine
Division of Cardiology
Department of Medicine
Medical University of South Carolina
Charleston, South Carolina

Reviewers

Linda Blust, MD
Assistant Professor of Internal Medicine
Medical College of Wisconsin
Milwaukee, Wisconsin

Laura J. Collins, MD
Internal Medicine
IOA/OnLok Senior Health
San Francisco, California

Ruth L. B. Ellen
4th Year Medical Student
University of Ottawa
Department of Internal Medicine
Ottawa, Canada

Charles Galaviz, MD
CA-1 in Anesthesia
The University of Iowa Hospitals and Clinics
Iowa City, Iowa

Michelle Grant Ervin, MD, MHPE, FACEP
Professor
Howard University
Washington, DC

Joe Hamilton, EMT-P, PA
National Health Service Corps (NHSC) Scholar
National Health Services, Inc.
Kern County, California

Jennifer Heidmann, MD
4th Year Resident
University of California at San Francisco
San Francisco, California

Rick Jotani, MD
1st Year Resident
Spartanburg Family Medicine Residency Program
Spartanburg, South Carolina

Brendan Kelley
4th Year Medical Student
Ohio State University
Columbus, Ohio

Alexandru F. Kimel
3rd Year Medical Student
New York Medical College—5th Pathway
Valhalla, New York

Lawrence Kirk Bennett
3rd Year Medical Student
President: Family Medicine Interest Group
Medical University of South Carolina College of Medicine
Charleston, South Carolina

Rachel Langland, MD
3rd Year Resident
St. Josephs Family Practice Residency Program
Phoenix, Arizona

Atif Malik, MD
Chief Resident
Department of PM & R
Baylor College of Medicine & UT Medical School
Houston, Texas

Amy Mohler, MD
1st Year Geriatric Fellow
Good Samaritan Regional Medical Center
Phoenix, Arizona

Gregory P. Schaefer
4th Year Medical Student
Lake Erie College of Osteopathic Medicine
Erie, Pennsylvania

Mark Watkins
4th Year Medical Student
Meharry Medical College
Nashville, Tennessee

Wendy L. Wright
3rd Year Medical Student
Meharry Medical College
Nashville, Tennessee

1

Palliation for Chronic Illness

George J. Taylor, Jerome E. Kurent,
John E. Heffner, and Frank J. Brescia

At the beginning of the twentieth century, 90% of deaths were from acute illnesses. Now 90% of patients die from a chronic disease, with about half receiving treatment for at least 30 months before they die (1). This means that most people have time to plan for end-of-life care.

There has been dissatisfaction with the quality of medical care at the end of life. Patients and their families often feel they cannot rely on their doctors or the health care system to control symptoms or follow their wishes. A common experience is that terminal care is delivered with confusion by a system that seems disinterested in this aspect of medical care. Energy may be expended—usually in the form of diagnostic studies aimed at new symptoms—but symptom control is inadequate. The patient may be told that nothing can be done for a significant complaint because it is an inevitable and untreatable symptom of the disease, a part of its natural history.

Doctors and other caregivers are not doing well either. Care of the dying is a major stress to clinicians who often report a sense of "suffering" while treating their dying patients (2). They experience feelings of frustration, helplessness, failure, uselessness, loneliness, or disappointment, while having an increased awareness of their own vulnerability and mortality. Factors that exacerbate physician distress in caring for the dying may include fear of dying, inadequate training, poor communication skills, conflicts regarding goals of care, unrealistic expectations, and uncertainty about treatment. On the other hand, physicians who treat the dying in palliative care settings are less conflicted than general practitioners who are involved with this aspect of patient care on only an occasional basis.

The care of dying patients has been a special reponsibility of the physician since antiquity. Helping people negotiate life's final transition should be rewarding, and it is when it is done well. The premise of this text is that sound clinical judgment and compassion regarding end-of-life planning and decision-making, plus skill with palliation and counseling will allow you to do great good, and will make this aspect of medicine especially rewarding.

A Good Death, Another Goal of Medicine

When dealing with an individual patient's problem it helps to think of the goals of care. For most of our lives, improved longevity is the primary goal. That has been the major thrust of scientific medicine, and all new treatments are tested for their effects on survival. A second goal of medicine, important at all stages of our lives, is the control of symptoms, which maximizes the quality of life.

A third goal, seldom discussed on the wards, is a good death. A peaceful death includes optimal control of pain and other symptoms, being in a comfortable setting (the preferred place of death is home for some, the hospital for others), and having family and friends present. Equally important, it means having adequate preparation so that anxiety and confusion are minimized, and that family, social, and spiritual affairs are in order. The spiritual dimensions of end-of-life care are increasingly recognized as being of critical importance for most terminally-ill patients.

In our personal lives, when considering our families or ourselves, we all would agree on the desirability of such a "good death." Unfortunately, doctors who have been trained that extending life is the standard by which their professional efforts will be judged frequently promote actions that make a peaceful death unlikely.

Have you noticed how doctors occasionally seem uncomfortable or embarrassed after the death of a patient? This may be apparent during discussions of "what went wrong" following an unsuccessful resuscitation effort in the intensive care unit. One reason for unease is that a terminally-ill patient may not be so identified, and care is not organized for the purpose of palliation and a peaceful death. Death may therefore be perceived as a failure.

We wince at the spectacle of the hopelessly-ill elderly person or the patient nearing the end of an obviously fatal illness who is subjected to a prolonged intensive care unit death, or the chronically-ill nursing home patient who is given tube feedings, yet both are common. No one feels good about it; not the doctor, not the family, and certainly not the patient. In contrast, when all have decided that the goal of care is a peaceful death, treating a patient at the end of life is a positive and rewarding clinical experience. For the patient and family it may be a time of spiritual growth.

When death is imminent, the doctor does not "give up" on the patient. On the contrary, the effective clinician appreciates the nature of distress, the meaning of suffering and is committed to "comfort always." The process leading to death must be made more humane, and the doctor works diligently to control symptoms, to provide counsel and to comfort. When done well, this includes an interdisciplinary team of trained caregivers; the good news is that the doctor is not in this alone. Furthermore, we are practicing at a time of increased interest in end-of-life care (3).

Medical Ethics and End-of-Life Care

During the last 3 decades, practice standards have shifted in favor of patient autonomy. Previously, the central ethic in the practice of medicine was beneficence: the all-knowing and beneficent physician was trusted to know, and then to do, what was in the patient's best interest. With this paternalistic model, the physician could view the patient as a passive recipient of care. Disagreeing with the doctor was considered inappropriate. (We all know doctors who continue to view any disagreement as an affront to their authority.)

The change to a patient autonomy model does not minimize the moral responsibility of the physician. Rather, the doctor's unquestioned control over what happens to the patient has been altered. Now the emphasis is on your obligation to inform, to carefully discuss alternatives, and then to respect and support the patient's wishes. What this means to all of us, as future patients, is that when we are sick we retain control of decision-making. That is what we want for our families and ourselves, and it should be what we offer to our patients.

The principle of non-maleficence is another ethical concept that should be kept in mind. "Do nothing to others you would not have done to you" has been identified as a reliable ethical test by many of the world's religions and by secular ethics as well (4). We are correct to advise medical students and young doctors to apply this test and to trust their instincts. If what they see happening to a patient seems wrong and not what they would allow for themselves or a family member, then it may well be wrong.

There are other ethical issues we face when caring for dying patients. The ethical principle of distributive justice recognizes that society has finite resources, and that financial and human resources are not limitless. Although we tend to make decisions based exclusively on the patient's best interest, there is no doubt that society also requires that we be good stewards. The principle of truth-telling indicates a moral and ethical obligation for the physician to provide all meaningful information to the patient in order to facilitate informed decision-making.

End-of-Life Decisions

Our initial reaction to critically ill patients is to save them. We are trained to prolong life, and aggressive therapy may work. But at what cost? An elderly person, or one with a severe life-limiting debilitating illness, may object that invasive interventions are not worth the cost in financial terms or personal suffering. The young doctor then points to Medicare and supplemental insurance and argues, "It is paid for."

The patient usually is referring to a different cost burden. Suffering is another expense. An octogenarian may realize that there is limited time ahead and knows that with the frailty of advanced age the recovery time from surgery is prolonged and the morbidity, higher. The decision that a small increment in survival is not worth what must be endured to purchase it can be a rational one. An insightful patient may perceive that "prolonging life" may instead mean "prolonging the dying process."

Whether to choose life-prolonging treatment is thus a value decision. It involves the patient's assessment of the probable quality of extra time, as well as all the "costs" of therapy. No one is qualified to make those value decisions for another person (certainly not the doctor).

A survey of elderly patients and their families has documented concern about inappropriate and aggressive care at the end of life (5). Subjects of the study felt they often were advised to choose procedures or an aggressive course of treatment they did not want. The best solution to the elderly or chronically-ill person's dilemma is adherence to the principle of autonomy, including a willingness of the doctor to accept and support a patient's decision to choose palliation when cure is no longer possible. You may feel that the patient has decided to give up too early and stands to lose years of good life unnecessarily. You can point this out, and it is your duty to give your best professional advice. But as you discharge this clinical responsibility, remember that you have nothing to "sell," and you must stop short of applying pressure. It is the informed patient's ultimate right to refuse therapy, even when you believe it may be a mistake to do so.

Such decisions are not always straightforward. A patient may decide that it is easier to die of heart disease than some other degenerative illness of old age. A survey of the families of 18,000 people who died after age 65 found that only 14% were fully functional in the last year of life (6). Most of the natural causes of death were preceded by disability and dependency. A prominent exception was death from acute myocardial infarction, where older patients "were far more likely to be fully functional in the year before death" (6).

Another example of choices is presented by a recent trial showing that implanted defibrillator therapy conveys a survival benefit to patients who have had myocardial infarction and left ventricular dysfunction by preventing death from ventricular fibrillation. However, those treated were more likely to die with congestive heart failure. Thus, a patient with advanced cardiac injury must choose between sudden cardiac death and somewhat longer survival but an uncomfortable death with associated pump failure (7).

Many illnesses that were once incurable are now easily cured. Unfortunately, what remains are conditions like dementia, stroke, heart failure, end-stage renal disease, and chronic neurological diseases. Because of the autonomy principle we may see an evolution in attitudes about end-of-life care. Presently, there is bias for prolonging life whenever it can be accomplished, even when quality of life may be poor (e.g., antibiotic therapy for urinary tract infection or tube feeding for a patient with advanced dementia).

How will attitudes about end-of-life care evolve?—Attitudes about dying and end-of-life care are basic cultural and societal issues. They may be expected to change slowly. Dissatisfaction with modern medicine's management at the end of life is one explanation for the *right to die* and physician assisted suicide movements. (A discussion of these subjects is beyond the scope of this book.)

An alternative would be to adopt a palliative model of care earlier in the course of an illness than is now customarily applied. Using the autonomy principle, a person who is experiencing decline and feels that the end of life is near may decide to "let nature take its course," with advance directives in place to decline treatment of illnesses like pneumonia. That decision would represent a "time-tradeoff": improving the odds for a rapid, natural, and peaceful death versus the risk of losing some period of useful life.

Currently, a person with decision-making capacity has the right to make that decision, just as there is a right to refuse life-prolonging chemotherapy or surgical repair of an aortic aneurysm. But in practice, many physicians would be uncomfortable withholding treatment of an easily cured infection.

Do not mistake this discussion as an argument against life-prolonging therapy for the elderly. That is not our intent, and we believe that age should *not* disqualify a person for any treatment. Treatment shown to prolong meaningful high quality life should be applied irrespective of age, *if that is what the patient wants.* Instead, our purpose—and yours—should be to support the patient who has decided to avoid life-prolonging and *unwanted* treatment.

The reverse side of this argument—The preceding discussion assumes that the patient chooses palliation rather than aggressive, life-prolonging care at the end of life. Equally common is the patient who wants to pursue a "cure," even when that is not possible, and when attempts to do so involves excessive suffering. The following are reasons that hinder the referral of patients to palliative services, such as hospice, even when it would be appropriate. You can see that errors in judgment may originate with care providers, the patient, or the family:

▶ The patient refuses to accept that cure is no longer possible.
▶ The patient understands, but family members are unable to face reality and insist on life-prolonging care.
▶ They deny the reality of the clinical prognosis.
▶ They believe the patient may qualify for a clinical research trial providing a miracle drug.
▶ The physician has either implied or stated unrealistic expectations about improved survival, symptoms, or quality of life.
▶ There is a perceived need to instill "hope" by treating and doing "something."
▶ The patients may distrust all medical care including hospice care and choose "alternative" medicine or unorthodox treatment.
▶ The patient may have strong religious beliefs that foresee cure if treatment is given. Perhaps there is hope for a miracle.

▶ Family caregivers resist hospice because it may replace the traditional role of family in caring for the dying family member.

When practicing medicine, we attempt what is clinically indicated, and when something fails, we stop. Patients may suffer because the doctor does not provide an adequate therapeutic trial, or because of persistence with futile procedures and treatments.

Determining futility is a dynamic process and involves critical decision-making that at times struggles between doing what is best for the patient and what the patient wants. We agree that there will always be an element of uncertainty when determining what is futile. Futility means different things to different people, and an absolute definition is difficult to apply. At the same time clinical reality demands choices, and doctors cannot be obligated to honor requests for treatment they consider useless or unethical.

Ethical issues that may be encountered when treating the dying patient are listed in Box 1-1 (and the list is not complete). A more thorough discussion is not possible in this introductory text.

The Physician's Role

Communicating: how to give bad news

The most difficult time to make end-of-life decisions is during an acute illness. It is hard for a patient and family to make rational choices in the face of distressing symptoms. Often they are dealing with an unfamiliar doctor in disorienting settings like the emergency room or the intensive care unit.

Instead, decisions about the goals and limits of medical care are best made when the patient with a chronic illness is stable and not in a crisis. The primary care practitioner is in the ideal position to initiate this process, as there is often a long history of a mutually rewarding patient-doctor relationship. Most patients expect their doctor to initiate discussion of advance care planning. The conversation may take place and decisions made over the course of several office visits. This provides the patient and family ample time to understand as much as possible about the illness, including the possibility of adverse clinical developments.

The first goal of these discussions is to educate the patient and family about the illness. Most diseases can be described in terms that a layperson can understand. You will be more effective if you are sitting at eye level with the patient. Do not assume medical sophistication, regardless of the person's level of education. Even those with advanced degrees may be confused about what the

BOX
1-1
| *Practical issues at the end of life that have ethical implications*

1. Truth-telling and prognosis: Should the patient be told bad news if he or she does not request the information? What do you do when the family asks that information be withheld (so the patient does not give up hope)?
2. When is death reasonable for a particular patient? How does the doctor know that further attempts at cure are futile?
3. How might definitions of futility vary among the patient, family, doctor, and society?
4. How is decision-making shared among patient, family, and physician? Often the family (or doctor) urges the patient to try anything, "not to give up."
5. Determining the patient's capacity to make decisions: When does the surrogate take over?
6. Patient participation in failing clinical trials. Does the doctor have a vested interest in the study?
7. Are food and hydration medical interventions? Should they be forced on the patient? (See Chapter 11.)
8. Escalation of analgesic doses for control of terminal symptoms: Might this hasten death, and is this euthanasia?
9. Treating pain in patients with a history of drug abuse or addiction.
10. When is enough, enough? What is enough? (Blood, parenteral nutrition, antibiotics, resuscitation, etc.)
11. How do you respond to requests for alternative, complementary, or unorthodox care?
12. How do you respond to the suicidal patient or one requesting assisted suicide?

kidneys or liver do. Patients are grateful when told how each medicine works, as well as the side effects that may be anticipated.

For a patient contemplating palliative care, the emphasis should be on the total care plan and what *will be done to control symptoms.* In this context limits of care can be decided. When not under pressure, all stakeholders can make their positions known. Including family caregivers in the decision process is critical, especially those who will eventually be surrogate decision-makers.

Patients and families may want medically sophisticated friends or relatives included in discussions, and that should be welcomed. The goals are to transmit information, instill trust, and to arrive at good decisions that reflect the patient's wishes. Anyone who can help you achieve these goals should be included (with the patient's permission). It may be helpful to schedule a "family conference." This forum has a number of advantages: it is an efficient way to communicate information to all of the interested parties, it carries the weight and gravity of a formal meeting, and as such, it emphasizes the doctor's concern and commitment.

Some of the following chapters provide sample conversations or guides for discussions with patients. These are not scripts to be memorized and delivered after taking a deep breath, but instead are intended as guides that can be adapted to your patient's circumstance and personality—and to yours.

Many of the sample conversations provide "openers" that facilitate the discussion of end-of-life issues. The best of these are questions. An especially useful question is "What is your understanding of the situation now?" This is not a "test" you are asking the patient or family to take, but instead is a request for information that will insure that you are all on the same wavelength. As is often the case, good communication begins with listening. Ideally, your time with the patient and family will involve dialogue, not monologue.

As part of the ongoing dialogue, the doctor should value contributions from nonfamily caregivers, especially those who are spending a lot of time with the patient. Many people find it easier to raise end-of-life concerns with a home health nurse, a social worker, a pulmonary rehabilitation nurse, or another who has frequent contact. Although final planning must include the doctor, any effort that gets the process started is welcome.

The role of the consultant

A subspecialist consultant may be asked to clarify specific clinical issues. It is important to select a sensible and experienced consultant, one who does not have a reputation for bending patients to his or her will. We are concerned that subspecialists tend to focus on the illness rather than the patient, and may feel an obligation to advocate for a potentially curative procedure (i.e., aortic valve replacement for an 85-year-old patient who does not want surgery). Primary care doctors may suffer from the same shortcoming, but at least the primary care doctor has usually had a longer experience with the patient as a person. Palliative care consultation is increasingly available in the United States, and is already well established in the United Kingdom where palliative medicine is considered a medical specialty.

Other tasks for the physician

As noted above, the doctor is the educator, responsible for helping the patient and family understand the illness and potential therapies. In many cases, a decision to avoid aggressive curative or life-prolonging therapy follows an understanding of its associated morbidity versus a slim chance for success. As a young doctor it is useful to pay attention to how physicians with more experience talk with patients and families. You will observe that those who are successful in practice usually have a reputation for explaining things well, being "the doctor who will talk with you."

Nonmedical people are concerned about how to act and what to do. We all fear behaving inappropriately, a real possibility in unfamiliar surroundings and in times of crisis. The doctor is able to tell the patient and family where to be, what to expect, what decisions may need to be made, and what the choices are.

The doctor is the one individual at the center of the illness who is not emotionally involved or grief-stricken. It is often a relief to have someone to turn to for straight talk, who is sympathetic, but is not sorrowful. Though dispassionate, the doctor is also a major source of comfort. The doctor has "been through it" with the patient and family, and is in a special position to comfort. Whether we like it or not, the white coat is a powerful robe of office. Even when we physicians are patients, we consider our doctors special (at least we need for them to be special).

A sympathetic word and a willingness to listen go a long way. If you sense that the patient needs to talk about more than just the illness, how do you start? An experienced teacher once suggested this phrase: "It's tough, isn't it?" That invitation usually works if the patient wishes to explore feelings and not strictly medical issues.

Patients commonly experience a fear of abandonment when facing terminal illness. They note a reluctance of family and friends to discuss the illness or the possibility of death. These are alien subjects, and your counsel may promote communication in the family. It is especially reassuring when you declare that you will be with the patient until the end. At the same time emphasize your commitment to good control of pain and other symptoms.

As an aside, the doctor continues to have responsibility after the patient dies. What you do is an important first step in bereavement counseling. If possible, meet with the family to review the medical issues, and to answer questions. Invite the family to contact you in the future if new questions arise. Most hospice organizations also provide post-death grief support for surviving family members.

A *letter of condolence* should be a part of your routine care (8). Even when you have already talked with the family, this formal expression is gratefully received. Furthermore, not communicating with the family may convey a lack of concern about their loss, even though you do not feel this. Some doctors worry that expressions of sorrow may be construed as a statement of guilt. If that is a consideration, use "I wish" rather than "I am sorry" (e.g., "I wish that Mr. Jones, you, and your family had not gone through this hard time") (9). In this note you should be truthful, and you should not say anything you do not mean. You might touch on your personal relationship with the patient (e.g., "I felt that Mr. Jones and I became friends during this time, and I will miss seeing him"). If it has been the case, comment on the faithful care provided by the spouse or family (e.g., "I was impressed by the way you stuck by him this last month, and expect it will be a source of comfort and satisfaction as you reflect on this experience").

Who is in control?

It is helpful to recognize the limitations of the physician. Doctors, particularly those with limited experience, often overestimate their influence at the end of life. Patients who are in intensive care units may be dependent on life-support devices, and withdrawal could result in death. In such cases, and in so many words, doctors have been known to say, "the patient only dies when I allow it." If this logic is pursued, the doctor is claiming control over life and death, a patently false notion.

Claiming control also suggests that the doctor has more responsibility for death than is the case. In matter of fact, a terminally-ill patient *dies of a disease*. To choose a metaphor, Mother Nature is in control. Our interventions may affect only the timing of death and the duration and extent of suffering. By withdrawing life-prolonging support at the patient's direction, the doctor is not responsible for causing death, nor is the patient. This is not considered physician assisted suicide or euthanasia. (Daniel Callahan develops this line of reasoning in *The Troubled Dream of Life* (10). We recommend it for you as well as your patients. It has been useful as a focus for community-based study groups.)

Advance Directives

Two documents are currently used, the living will and durable power of attorney for health care. It is unnecessary to have both, and a durable power of attorney for health care is the more powerful and useful instrument, as it names and empowers a decision-maker in the event there is a loss of decision-making capacity (11). It is generally advised not to have both documents concurrently, as they may come into conflict with each other.

In its weakest form, the living will is a general document, providing a general guide such as "I do not wish aggressive or heroic measures if there is little chance for success." This leaves much room for interpretation. Specific instructions are more useful. Living will statutes may vary somewhat from state to state, but the spirit and intent of this document are similar. Advise your patients to be as specific as possible. Most living wills also have provisions for care in the event of persistent vegetative state (PVS). Even though most people would not anticipate experiencing PVS, it is advisable to provide advance instructions for this albeit unlikely circumstance.

A patient with advanced lung disease who does not want future ventilator support may indicate this in the living will. Similarly, an elderly person with severe life-limiting disability could declare a choice of palliation over cure for acute illnesses. This might include avoiding antibiotics for infections like pneumonia or urosepsis. Provisions can be written to withdraw ventilator support if a determination is made that no meaningful recovery is possible.

Instructions to avoid tube feeding for a patient with advanced dementia can also be provided by a durable power of attorney document or living will. Advance directives are legal documents, and a family member or the physician cannot overrule the living will.

A living will is unnecessary when a durable power of attorney for health care has named a surrogate decision-maker (11). When the patient is not competent, the surrogate is assumed to speak with the patient's voice. Thus, the surrogate is empowered to make a decision about care even if it appears to conflict with the living will. The surrogate must feel secure with knowledge of the patient's desires. It is advisable for some of the discussion between surrogate and patient to include the primary care physician and other family members.

One problem with the living will is that it may not cover some clinical circumstances, however detailed and specific it may be. A surrogate is able to address any eventuality, using the patient's general wishes as a guide. There may even be an implicit wish for the doctor and surrogate to overrule the general provisions of a living will if unusual clinical circumstances develop. At the point the patient is unable to make decisions there is an obvious loss of autonomy, and the surrogate and doctor are expected to respect the patient's wishes.

Planning end-of-life care becomes less about selecting from a menu of desirable life-sustaining interventions, and is more important as a statement about comprehensive life goals. These goals, from the patient's perspective, center on preparing for a dignified death, achieving a level of spiritual peace, having some control over the dying process, strengthening personal relationships with family and friends, and saying final good byes. Physicians tend to see advance care planning as a process that selects treatment interventions. Patients see end-of-life planning as a broader process that also addresses psychological, emotional, and spiritual goals—as well as treatment preferences and avoidances.

Hospice Care and Principles of Palliative Care

Palliative medicine is not a novel issue. Principles of palliative care have recently been enumerated, and are as listed in Box 1-2. They describe what care can and should be like for everyone facing the end of life. Palliative care affirms life, and regards dying as a normal process; it neither hastens nor postpones death; it provides relief from pain and other distressing symptoms; it integrates the psychological and spiritual aspects of patient care; and it offers a support system to help the family cope during the patient's illness and with their own bereavement.

The hospice Medicare benefit is the most commonly utilized model for providing palliative care, and has been in existence since 1982 (12). The United States began the 1970s without a certified hospice, until 1974 when a home care program opened in New Haven, Connecticut. In 1980, the government funded 26 demonstration hospice projects to evaluate the quality of care, utilization of services, and costs. There was obvious

BOX 1-2	*Five principles of palliative care*

1. Palliative care respects the goals, likes, and choices of the dying person.
2. Palliative care looks after the medical, emotional, social, and spiritual needs of the dying person.
3. Palliative care supports the needs of the family.
4. Palliative care helps gain access to needed health care providers and appropriate care settings.
5. Palliative care builds ways to provide excellent care at the end of life.

political appeal to pass legislation when an estimated cost savings of $150 million by 4000 hospice patients was calculated in the early 1980s.

In 1983, hospice services became part of the Medicare benefits program featuring the following major components: (1) physician certified patient prognosis of 6 months or less; (2) a payment cap on in-patient hospice service to encourage home care utilization; (3) revocation of all other Medicare benefits; (4) spiritual, bereavement, and volunteer services mandated for each program reimbursed on a per diem basis; (5) drug prescription benefit for medications and palliative procedures; (6) attending physician billing services thru Medicare Part B.

By 2000 there were more than 3000 hospice programs in the United States treating an estimated 700,000 patients (1). Medicare is the source of payment for 65% of them. The mean length of hospice service days has changed dramatically, from 70 days in 1983 to 36 days in 1999 (13). This reduction in length of time patients are in hospice before dying suggests that we presently initiate palliative care too late in the course of chronic illness.

What hospice means to your patient—When discussing hospice care with your patient, clearly state what hospice is and does. First, in the United States hospice is not a physical location for patients to be taken to die. This is an unfortunate misconception of many patients. Instead, the hospice Medicare benefit is interdisciplinary home-based care. The usual experience is that hospice gathers the patient and family in and makes everything better.

Some terminally-ill patients avoid enrolling in hospice because it implies "giving up." Avoid telling your patient, "There is nothing more I can do for you, so I am sending you to hospice." Hospice in fact represents comprehensive supportive care designed to maximize quality of life at the end of life.

A hospice interdisciplinary care team provides services including nursing care, pain and symptom management, spiritual support, anticipatory and after-death grief support, and caregiver support. The team includes hospice nurses and nursing aides, a social worker, a chaplain, and a physician medical director. Hospice also relies heavily on carefully trained volunteers who provide help of all kinds: visiting with the patient and family, helping with shopping, providing transportation when needed, dealing with pets, simple home repairs—whatever needs to be done. In this context, the patient and family are considered the care unit. It is important for them to realize that hospice supports the family, but does not replace its traditional role.

The patient and family quickly realize that the hospice nurse is the key person on the team. The nurse visits 2 or 3 times a week, or more depending on specific needs. Hospice nurses tend to be especially skillful. They are expert with medicines used to treat pain and other symptoms, and with managing their side effects. In addition to scheduled visits, most hospices are organized to respond to emergencies at night and on weekends. The nature of hospice nursing selects people who are competent, kind and mature, who are dedicated to caring for terminally-ill patients, and who are able to operate independently.

In addition to home services, the hospice benefit provides for brief hospital admissions for "respite." This gives the family caregivers a chance to rest. In addition, short periods of hospitalization, either in a freestanding hospice unit, nursing home, or the hospital, are covered for adjusting therapy if this has not been possible at home.

How hospice works for the doctor—The doctor who refers a patient to hospice may continue managing the patient's illness, and does not relinquish the care of the patient. The hospice medical director, a physician, functions as an informal consultant and as support for the hospice team. In actual practice, the patient's physician determines the medical director's level of involvement. When that doctor is closely involved, the hospice physician remains in the background, a "silent partner." If, for whatever reason, the patient's doctor is not involved, the hospice physician is able to step in and help.

Eligibility and enrollment in hospice—Most patients enrolled in hospice have a diagnosis of cancer, but there are increasing numbers of patients with non-cancer diagnoses. These include end-stage congestive heart failure, advanced lung disease, end-stage neurologic diseases such as amyotrophic lateral sclerosis and Alzheimer's disease, AIDS, end-stage renal disease, and other terminal conditions. To qualify a patient must have a life expectancy of 6 months or less, as estimated by the patient's physician. However, if the patient survives beyond that period, the hospice benefit may be extended.

While Medicare is the prevailing model of hospice care in the United States, private insurers also provide this benefit. Other models are also evolving such as hospital-based palliative care services which may interface closely with hospice.

Cultural Influences on End-of-Life Care

Ethnic and cultural diversity has significant impact on preferences at the end of life. Preferences for life-prolonging interventions, and preferred place of death may vary by ethnic and cultural heritage. Rituals regarding care of the recently deceased patient have significant implications for the caregiver. Hospice may be perceived by some as potentially displacing the role of the family.

A family's religious beliefs may influence end-of-life decisions. We are unaware of any faith tradition that places limits on control of pain and other distressing symptoms for terminally-ill patients. Other medical decisions may be affected (i.e., avoidance of blood products by Jehovah's witnesses). A thorough review of this important subject is beyond the scope of this introductory text.

The Last Hours: Managing Symptoms in the Terminal Patient

Signs and symptoms of imminent death may lead the patient or family to request or demand hospitalization. Many assume that dying at home is always better and easier than in the hospital, but that is not true for all patients. Those who have been treated in hospice are usually comfortable with death at home. Without hospice support, many families are not prepared to treat a terminally-ill patient during the last hours of life. Nursing services in acute care hospitals do a good job managing terminal symptoms when "comfort care" is clearly identified as the goal of treatment. However, there is the risk that a terminally-ill patient could receive inappropriate and aggressive interventions if the medical team is not fully informed of the care plan for terminal care.

Symptoms often escalate in the hours just before death. In fact, an abrupt increase in symptoms that had been previously controlled often signals that death is imminent. This can be especially distressing to the patient and family. Increasing the dose of analgesics may help, but at doses that may further compromise cognition and the ability to communicate. The "death rattle" due to the patient's inability to clear loose upper airway secretions may be alarming to family caregivers who may benefit from discussion provided by trained professionals, such as hospice personnel.

The trade-off between terminal symptom control and consciousness can sometimes be difficult to negotiate. The patient and/or family should guide therapy, preferable in advance of the active dying process. When discomfort is severe, they will demand relief and you must not hesitate to provide appropriate care.

Higher dose opioids may be titrated to relieve symptoms whether for treatment of pain or dyspnea. Though unusual in the patient on chronic opioid therapy, there may be depression of respiration with higher doses necessary to provide adequate relief of terminal symptoms. In this case the ethical imperative is to help your dying patient who is suffering, even if high-dose opioids contributes to an earlier death. There is no culpability. This is not assisted suicide or euthanasia, but rather necessary treatment of extreme symptoms (using the language of ethicists, a "choice of the greater good") (14). It is, however, important that if this approach is utilized, that the decision be made in collaboration with the patient or surrogate decision-maker.

References

1. Guyer B, Freedman MA, Strobino DM, Sondik EJ. Annual summary of vital statistics; trends in the health of Americans in the 20th century. Pediatrics 2000;106:1307–1317.

2. Cherny NI, Catane R. Palliative medicine and the medical oncologist. Defining the purview of care. Hematol Oncol Clin North Am 1996;10:1–20.

3. SUPPORT Investigators. A controlled trial to improve care for seriously ill hospitalized patients. The study to understand prognosis and

preferences for outcomes and risks of treatments (SUPPORT). JAMA 1995;274:1591–1598.

4. Singer P. Practical Ethics. Cambridge: Cambridge University Press, 1979.

5. Lynn J, Teno JM, Phillips RS, et al. Perceptions by family members of the dying experience of older and seriously ill patients. Ann Intern Med 1997;126:97–102.

6. Lentzner H, Pamuk E, Rhodenhiser, et al. The quality of life in the year before death. Am J Public Health 1992;82:1093–1099.

7. Moss AJ, Zareba W, Hall WJ, et al. Prophylactic implantation of a defibrillator in patients with myocardial infarction and reduce ejection fraction. N Engl J Med 2002;346:877–883.

8. Bedell SE, Cadenhead K, Graboys TB. The doctor's letter of condolence. N Engl J Med 2001;344:1162–1163.

9. Quill TE, Arnold RM, Platt F. "I wish things were different": expressing wishes in response to loss, futility, and unrealistic hopes. Ann Intern Med 2001;135:551–555.

10. Callahan D. The Troubled Dream of Life. New York: Simon & Schuster, 1993.

11. Menikoff JA, Sachs GA, Siegler M. Beyond advance directives—health care surrogate laws. N Engl J Med 1992;327:1165–1168.

12. Bayer R, Feldman E. Hospice under the medicare wing. Hastings Cent Rep 1982;12:5–9.

13. Christakis N, Lamont E. Extent and determinants of error in doctors' prognoses in terminally ill patients: prospective cohort study. BMJ 2000;320:469–476.

14. Sachs GA, Ahronheim JC, Rhymes JA, et al. Good care of dying patients: the alternative to physician-assisted suicide and euthanasia. J Am Geriatr Soc 1995;43:553–556.

2

The Pharmacology of Symptom Control

Kristi L. Lenz

Pain Control

Fear of pain and the fear of dying in pain are among the greatest concerns of patients near the end of life (1,2). On the other hand, control of most pain in a palliative care setting is fairly easily achieved when clinicians know the basic principles of pain management and understand how to use analgesics.

There are barriers to good pain control. Patients, their families, and doctors may be reluctant to use medicines with possible side effects. Media representation of the risks of opioids contributes to this; recent stories have focused on possible addiction, and there have been malpractice suits in such cases. The most effective drugs are controlled substances, and concern about regulatory review is intimidating. Nevertheless, when treating patients at the end of life, our responsibility is adequate palliation of symptoms, a prerequisite for a peaceful death.

The most common error in practice is the failure to prescribe doses adequate to control symptoms. Box 2-1 outlines general principles of pain management, and provides a framework for the more detailed discussion that follows.

Non-opioid Analgesics

Pharmacology and dosing

Non-opioid analgesics include aspirin (ASA), non-acetylated salicylates, non-steroidal anti-inflammatory drugs (NSAIDs), and acetaminophen (3). These agents are the drugs of choice for mild to moderate pain. All act peripherally to inhibit cyclooxygenase, which converts arachadonic acid to prostaglandins.

Prostaglandins sensitize nociceptive neurons; therefore, inhibition decreases pain transmission. Non-opioids are particularly effective for inflammatory pain. Acetaminophen is a weaker inhibitor of cyclooxygenase with less anti-inflammatory action. However, it is often used because of its limited adverse effect profile.

| BOX 2-1 | *Basic principles of pain management in the palliative care setting* |

Use Oral Agents Whenever Possible
Oral analgesics are the most cost-effective and convenient. They continue to work for the terminal patient: 60% of patients can take oral medications within 72 hours of death, and 20% within 24 hours of death.

Match the Analgesic to the Degree of Pain
Patients with mild to moderate pain may be started on a non-opioid or a combination product with a "weak" opioid. If pain progresses or is not controlled, a pure opioid agonist should be used (the non-opioid may be continued). Adjuvant agents should be used when appropriate at all levels of pain.

Administer Medications on a Scheduled Basis
It takes less medicine to prevent pain than to treat it. Start a regular schedule of medications, with doses gradually increased until the patient is comfortable. "As needed" or "PRN" dosing should be reserved for breakthrough doses and never as the sole means of pain relief in a patient with chronic pain.

Use Long-Acting Agents Whenever Possible
Sustained release (SR) products are much more convenient for patients than short-acting opioids taken at 3 hour intervals around the clock. The SR products are more expensive, and most manufacturers have assistance programs for medically indigent patients.

Use Appropriate Breakthrough Doses
"As needed" doses should be based upon the daily opioid dose, generally 10% to 20% of total daily dose. For example, if a patient is receiving SR morphine 100 mg twice daily, there should be an order for 30 mg of immediate-release morphine for breakthrough pain. Any short-acting opioid may be used, but morphine is the least expensive. Patients with high breakthrough doses may need concentrated solutions (morphine or oxycodone at 20 mg/mL) to avoid taking large numbers of tablets. Breakthrough opioids should be available at an appropriate interval, usually every 3 hours. Most short-acting opioids do not last more than 4 hours, so avoid the conventional "every 4 to 6 hours PRN pain."

Maximize Dose and Schedule Before Adding or Changing Drugs

It is inconvenient and illogical to have a patient on more than one SR product. Remember that opioids have no ceiling effect. Instead of adding an additional agent, simply increase the dose of the first. There is inter-patient variability in efficacy between opioids. If your patient is not obtaining pain relief at a high dose (or a dose causing side effects not easily controlled), try changing to a different drug.

Anticipate Adverse Effects

Counsel patients that nausea/vomiting and sedation are possible but that tolerance to these effects will occur in a few days. It is also very important to be proactive in anticipating and preventing opioid-induced constipation.

Evaluate Frequently

Patients on oral medications should initially be evaluated once or twice daily to assure breakthrough doses are adequate and that pain is controlled on SR products (this is an advantage of hospitalization when starting therapy). Patients with severe pain and those on IV opioids should be evaluated every few hours and the dose titrated upward appropriately. Ambulatory patients should be instructed to call you if they are using more than two breakthrough doses per day. This often indicates the need to increase the dose of their scheduled, long-acting agent.

Use Appropriate Adjuvant Agents

Particular types of pain respond best to adjuvant therapy (see text). Add these agents to opioids and titrate appropriately.

The most important principle to understand when using non-opioids for pain is that they have a "ceiling effect." There is a maximum daily dose above which there will be no increase in analgesia, but a substantial increase in adverse effects. With non-opioids there is no role, therefore, for pushing the dose beyond the manufacturer's recommended maximum. If a patient has persistent pain on the maximum dose of a non-opioid, an opioid analgesic should be added.

Available non-opioid agents and the usual doses are listed in Table 2-1. Over a dozen NSAIDs are available, as well as various salicylates and the newer cyclooxygenase-2 (COX-2) inhibitors. The potency and dosing intervals (and to a lesser degree, adverse effects) of these agents differ. However, no one is significantly

TABLE 2-1	*Non-Opioid Analgesics*

Generic Name	Trade Name	Usual Dose	Max Dose Per 24 Hours
Acetaminophen	Tylenol	325–650 mg PO Q4–6H	4000 mg
Salicylates			
Aspirin	Bayer	325–650 mg PO Q4–6H	6000 mg
Choline Mg salicylate	Trilisate	500–1500 mg PO Q8–12H	4500 mg
Diflunisal	Dolobid	250–500 mg PO Q8–12H	1500 mg
Salsalate	Disalcid	500–1500 mg PO Q8–12H	3000 mg
Propionic Acids			
Fenoprofen	Nalfon	300–600 mg PO Q6–8H	3200 mg
Flurbiprofen	Ansaid	50–100 mg PO Q8–12H	300 mg
Ibuprofen	Motrin	400–800 mg Q6–8H	3200 mg
Ketoprofen	Orudis	IR: 50–75 mg PO Q6–8H	300 mg
		SR: 100–200 mg PO QD	
Naproxen	Naprosyn	250–500 mg Q8–12H	1500 mg
Oxaprozin	Daypro	1200 mg PO QD	1800 mg
Acetic Acids			
Diclofenac	Voltaren	IR: 50–100 mg PO Q12H	200 mg
		SR: 100 mg PO QD	
with misoprostal	Arthrotec	50 mg/200 mg PO Q6–12H	
Etodolac	Lodine	200–400 mg PO Q6–12H	1200 mg
Indomethacin	Indocin	IR: 25–50 mg PO Q8–12H	IR: 200 mg
		SR: 75 mg PO Q12–24H	SR: 150 mg
Ketorolac	Toradol	PO: 10 mg PO Q4–6H	PO: 40 mg
		IV: 15–30 mg IV Q6H	IV: 120 mg
Nabumetone	Relafen	500–1000 mg PO QD	2000 mg
Sulindac	Clinoril	150–200 mg PO Q12H	400 mg
		300–400 mg PO QD	
Tolmetin	Tolectin	200–600 mg PO Q8H	1800 mg
Fenamates			
Meclofenamate	Meclomen	50–100 mg PO Q6–8H	400 mg
Mefenamic acid	Ponstel	250 mg PO Q6H	1000 mg
Oxicams			
Piroxicam	Feldene	10 mg PO Q12–24H	20 mg
COX-2 Inhibitors			
Celecoxib	Celebrex	100–200 mg PO BID	400 mg
Rofecoxib	Vioxx	12.5–50 mg PO QD	50 mg

PO = oral; IR = immediate-release; SR = sustained-release; IV = intravenous.

more effective than another, and the choice of an agent is primarily empiric. There does appear to be some variability of response, and when a patient does not respond to one type of non-opioid, you my have success switching to an agent in a different class. Non-opioids are synergistic with opioid analgesics, and the two classes are often used together.

Common adverse effects

Gastrointestinal effects—Gastrointestinal (GI) effects include nausea, vomiting, gastric irritation, and the risk of peptic ulcer disease (PUD) and are the most common adverse effects with aspirin and NSAIDs. Patients should be advised to take NSAIDs with food to minimize minor GI effects. The risk of PUD with long-term NSAID use is 1% after 3 to 6 months of use and 2% to 4% after 12 months of use. Patients at high risk of PUD (e.g., elderly patients, patients on concurrent anticoagulation) may be considered for ulcer prophylaxis with misoprostil. H2-antagonists (famotidine, ranitidine, cimetidine, nizatidine) have *not* been shown to be as effective as misoprostil at preventing NSAID-induced PUD.

The non-acetylated salicylates and acetaminophen have a minimal incidence of GI effects. The COX-2 inhibitors (celecoxib, rofecoxib) also appear to have a lower incidence of GI effects when compared to conventional NSAIDs; however, they are not devoid of this effect and are not considered appropriate substitutes for those at high risk for PUD.

Nephrotoxicity—Prostaglandins are renal vasodilators, and prostaglandin inhibition may cause a rise in serum creatinine. It may occur with all NSAIDs, including COX-2 inhibitors. Elderly patients are most susceptible, and in these patients, acetaminophen may be a better alternative. Persistent treatment with NSAIDs may lead to renal failure.

Hepatotoxicity—Liver injury is the primary concern with long-term use of acetaminophen. Patients with normal liver function may be safely given up to 4 grams per day on a chronic basis. Use caution in patients with underlying liver disease, and remember that most non-opioid/opioid combination products contain 325–500 mg of acetaminophen per tablet.

Anti-platelet effects—Aspirin has the most profound effect, inhibiting platelet aggregation for the life of the platelet (normally 7 to 10 days). Other NSAIDs cause reversible inhibition of platelet aggregation, with effects diminishing once the drug is cleared from the body. An anti-platelet effect is problematic when there is thrombocytopenia, concomitant warfarin therapy, or active bleeding. Non-acetylated salicylates, COX-2 inhibitors, and acetaminophen have minimal anti-platelet effects.

Central nervous system effects—These include tinnitus, dizziness, and confusion and are primarily seen with salicylates. The elderly are most susceptible to central nervous system (CNS) effects. A concern about CNS effects does not preclude the use of non-opioids. Just be aware of these possibilities, especially confusion in elderly patients.

Opioid Analgesics

Pharmacology and dosing

In the palliative care community, the term *opioid* is preferred to *narcotic*, as the latter has negative connotations implying an illegal or addictive drug. The site of action of opioid analgesics is centrally in the brain and spinal cord. All drugs in this class act at the same receptors and differ only with respect to potency (affinity for receptor subtypes), duration of action, and available routes of administration. All opioids are metabolized in the liver, and many have active metabolites that contribute to analgesia.

Opioid agonists have no ceiling effect. They are the drugs of choice for severe pain: that is the most important, basic concept in pain management. There is no maximum daily dose; the dose can always be increased to achieve analgesia. It is particularly important to explain this concept to patients who want to "save" these stronger drugs for the very end of life when pain may be severe. In practice, lower doses may be used early for less severe discomfort, and the dose raised to achieve good pain control as needed.

Table 2-2 lists available opioid agonists, with relative intravenous (IV) and oral potencies (4,5). Conversion from one of these drugs to another involves the formation of a simple ratio. For example, 30 mg of oral morphine is equal to 7.5 mg of oral hydromorphone (about a 4 : 1 conversion). Therefore, to achieve the same analgesia as 60 mg of oral morphine, about 10 mg of oral hydromorphone would need to be given. Keep in mind that these ratios are a reasonable place to start, but patient differences will require you to titrate the dose up or down based on response.

TABLE 2-2	*Equianalgesic Doses of Opioids**

Drug	Duration of Action	Equigesic IV Dose*	Equigesic PO Dose*
Codeine	3–4 hrs	130 mg	200 mg
Fentanyl**	IV: 1–3 hrs	0.1 mg	—
	patch: 48–72 hrs		
Hydrocodone	3–5 hrs	—	200 mg
Hydromorphone	2–3 hrs	1.5 mg	7.5 mg
Meperidine***	2–3 hrs	75 mg	300 mg
Methadone	6–8 hrs	acute: 10 mg	acute: 20 mg
		chronic: 2–4	chronic: 2–4 mg
Morphine	IR: 3–4 hrs	10 mg	acute: 60 mg
	SR: 8–24 hrs		chronic: 30 mg
Oxycodone	IR: 3–5 mg	—	20–30 mg
	SR: 12 hrs		
Propoxyphene	3–6 hrs	—	100–200 mg

IV = SC = IM doses and PO = PR doses; IR = immediate-release; SR = sustained-release.
* You may read this table vertically (by columns) or horizontally (by row); thus morphine 30 mg (given chronically) is roughly equivalent to 20 mg oxycodone.
** Fentanyl Patch: a 50 mcg/hr patch is roughly equivalent to IV morphine, 30 mg per day (and chronic oral morphine, 90 mg per day).
*** Meperidine is included for completeness. It is not recommended for chronic therapy, and thus has limited application in the palliative care setting.

When switching a patient from one opioid to another, consider starting with an equivalent dose that is lower (by 30% to 50%). The reason for this is variability among patients with respect to efficacy, adverse effects, and tolerance. If the initial response to the new drug is inadequate, the dose can be raised quickly.

Morphine—Morphine is the naturally occurring opioid, extracted from the opium poppy (*Papaver somniferum*). It is the standard by which other opioids and other analgesics are judged. In the absence of contraindications, morphine is the drug of choice for moderate to severe pain. There is no agent that is clinically superior to morphine. Furthermore, morphine has the most flexibility in dosing forms, is the most readily available, and is relatively inexpensive.

Morphine does have an active metabolite, morphine-6-glucuronide, that has analgesic action and has a half-life twice as long as the parent compound. It is eliminated renally, so use caution when administering morphine chronically in patients with renal insufficiency.

Single-dose studies demonstrate a 6:1 oral to IV ratio with morphine (Table 2-2). However, with repeated dosing, this ratio becomes 3:1, and this is the oral to IV ratio that should be used in the management of chronic pain.

Codeine—Codeine is also naturally occurring but is a weak opioid agonist. This means that at higher doses, adverse effects tend to overshadow gains in analgesia. We generally use codeine in combination with non-opioids for mild to moderate pain.

Fentanyl—This is a highly potent synthetic opioid that is lipophilic. This property means more rapid crossing of the blood-brain barrier (compared with hydrophilic agents like morphine). More important, a compound must be lipophilic for transdermal application.

The intravenous form of fentanyl is short acting (minutes) and is commonly used for acute perioperative pain management and conscious sedation. Fentanyl may be given by IV infusion for severe chronic pain, but it is more commonly prescribed as the transdermal patch (Duragesic). It is now available as a transmucosal lozenge for breakthrough pain. Because it is a synthetic product, fentanyl seems to cause less constipation and pruritus than morphine and codeine. Titration of patches during an acute pain crisis can be difficult because 12 to 24 hours are needed to achieve a steady state once a patch is applied. Ideally, patch doses should not be changed more often than every 1 to 2 days.

The best approach for patients with rapidly escalating pain is treatment with intravenous opioids to achieve control quickly, then conversion to the appropriate fentanyl patch dose. Dose conversions between fentanyl patches and other opioids have been reported in very wide ranges, and the manufacturer's recommendations are conservative. Our experience with a hospice population is that 30 mg of IV morphine per day is equivalent to a 50 mcg/hr fentanyl patch (changed every 72 hours).

Hydrocodone—This is a codeine derivative and another relatively weak opioid. It is given orally and is commonly used in combination with non-opioids for mild to moderate pain.

Hydromorphone—This is a semi-synthetic opioid derived from morphine. It has high potency, making it useful for concentrated intravenous or subcutaneous infusions. However, for long-term oral use, it is less useful than morphine. It is poorly absorbed (intravenous to oral ratio, 1:5), and there is no sustained-release formulation currently available.

Meperidine—Meperidine is a synthetic opioid in the same class as fentanyl. The usual use of this drug is the management of post-operative pain. It is seldom used for palliation of chronic pain because of poor oral absorption, a short duration of action, and the toxic metabolite, normeperidine. Normeperidine is eliminated by the kidneys and has a half-life four times longer than the parent compound (12 to 16 hours). In patients with renal dysfunction and those receiving high doses, accumulation of normeperidine may cause seizures or other CNS side effects. For this reason, the use of meperidine for chronic pain is discouraged.

Methadone—Like fentanyl and meperidine, methadone is a synthetic opioid. The duration of analgesia is 6 to 8 hours, considerably longer than others in the class. It also is well absorbed. Lower doses, under 50 mg per day, are safe and effective even when given for months. However, escalation to high dose therapy can be difficult because it has a pharmacokinetic half-life of 25 hours (much longer than the duration of analgesia). To avoid excessive accumulation, those on a maintenance dose of methadone should not use it for breakthrough pain. Instead, they should be provided with a short-acting opioid (e.g., morphine, hydromorphone) for breakthrough pain.

In practice, the long half-life makes the use of methadone for chronic pain management tricky. If you have little experience with it, methadone should not be your first choice. The caveat "start low and go slow" truly applies when converting patients from other opioids to methadone, as there is wide interpatient variability in response.

On the plus side, methadone is the cheapest opioid available, and many feel this earns it a place on the pain management roster. It may be unavailable for chronic pain in some states where it is restricted to methadone-maintenance programs (or may require special licensing).

Oxycodone—This is a semi-synthetic opioid derived from morphine. It is equipotent to oral morphine and is available both in combination with non-opioids, as well as "plain" in both immediate-release (IR) and sustained-release (SR) tablets. The SR form, OxyContin, is relatively easy to alter, and there has been abuse of the product (with the expected bad press). The manufacturer is re-formulating OxyContin to make abuse more difficult. Plain oxycodone is less commonly available than morphine in many community pharmacies. As it is short acting, it is good for breakthrough pain. An advantage of this drug, I have noticed, is that patients who attach a stigma to taking morphine often find oxycodone acceptable.

Propoxyphene—This is structurally similar to methadone and is a weak opioid. It is only available orally and is used in combination with aspirin or acetaminophen for mild pain. As with meperidine, the half-lives of propoxyphene and its metabolite, norpropoxyphene, are much longer than the duration of analgesia, leading to accumulation and CNS side effects with chronic therapy. The risk of this is highest with elderly patients. Propoxyphene offers no advantage over the other weak opioid combination products and should not be used for pain management in palliative care. In fact, some trials have shown no advantage of propoxyphene over aspirin.

Routes of administration

Opioid agonists can be administered by almost every route imaginable (Table 2-3). The choice of delivery system is highly dependent upon patient preference, anticipated duration of use, administration setting (inpatient versus outpatient), and the dose required for pain control. Morphine currently has the most flexibility in routes available, but new preparations of other drugs are being approved that will expand our choices.

Oral—This is preferred for chronic pain because of ease of administration, low rate of complications, and decreased cost. Absorption ("bioavailability") of opioid agonists differs greatly (Table 2-2), with hydromorphone the worst and methadone the best absorbed.

Onset of pain relief with immediate-release tablets and solutions is generally 30 to 60 minutes. If a more immediate effect is desired, opt for parenteral dosing. Also be certain to re-enforce correct doses with your patients when prescribing oral solutions, as both standard and concentrated solutions are available (e.g., morphine is available as 20 mg per 5 mL and as 20 mg per 1 mL).

A substantial advance in chronic pain management has been development of oral *SR preparations*. Both morphine and oxycodone are commercially available as twice daily (every 12 hours) dosing formulations, and SR hydromorphone has been submitted to the FDA for approval.

TABLE 2-3	*Opioid Agonist Preparations*			

Generic Name	Trade Name	Available IV?	Available PO?	Other Routes
Morphine	Kadian MS Contin Oramorph Roxanol	Yes	IR & SR tabs PO solutions	Suppositories
Codeine	—	Yes	IR tabs PO solutions	—
Fentanyl	Actiq Duragesic Sublimaze	Yes	No	Transmucosal lozenge; transdermal patch
Hydromorphone	Dilaudid	Yes	IR tabs PO solutions	Suppositories
Meperidine	Demerol	Yes	IR tabs PO solutions	—
Methadone*	Dolophine	Yes	IR tabs PO solutions	—
Oxycodone	OxyContin OxyFast Roxicodone	No	IR & SR tabs PO solutions	—
Propoxyphene	Darvon	No	IR caps PO solutions	—

IR = immediate-release; SR = sustained-release; SL = sublingual; PO = oral.
* Use methodone with caution because of a long and unpredictable half-life, especially in the elderly.

The SR tablets should not be crushed, as that destroys the SR effect. Kadian, a daily SR morphine capsule, may be opened and the granules emptied onto soft food for patients unable to swallow pills. None of SR products are easily administered through a percutaneous endoscopic gastrostomy (PEG) or jejunostomy tube (J-tube).

Although the SR opioids have an outstanding efficacy record, patients with *hepatic dysfunction* must use them with caution because of a limited ability to metabolize opioids. In this patient population, you may be able to use immediate-release products at extended intervals (e.g., every 6 or 8 hours).

Transdermal—The only opioid available for transdermal administration is fentanyl. Patches are applied every 72 hours and are convenient for patients not able to take oral tablets/capsules. The 3-day patch may help with medicine compliance in some cases. Advise patients to apply the patch over an area with adequate subcutaneous fat (e.g., chest wall, abdomen, upper arm, thigh) so that a depot of fentanyl may be formed. This route of administration is best used when patients have relatively stabilized pain. When converting patients on oral or IV opioids to fentanyl patches, be sure to continue the shorter-acting drug with a 24-hour overlap to account for the slow onset. Also, start with a lower dose patch.

A 100 mcg/hr fentanyl patch is currently the largest strength available, so patients needing higher doses will need to apply multiple patches. Practically, patients requiring more than three or four 100-mcg patches have difficulty finding enough adequate application sites, and should be considered for an alternate route (IV or subcutaneous infusion). When there are adverse effects, be aware that removal of the patches still leaves a 12 to 24 hour depot of drug in the subcutaneous tissue.

Buccal/Sublingual—This route is useful when a patient loses IV access and cannot swallow. Fentanyl has a buccal bioavailability of 50%, hydromorphone 25%, and morphine 20%. Morphine immediate-release tablets and the concentrated oral solution may be given sublingually, and a commercially available transmucosal fentanyl lozenge is also available (Actiq). The effective fentanyl lozenge dose is highly variable between patients, and the chronic opioid dose does not predict response. Therefore, patients should be started on the lowest dose (200 mcg lozenge) and titrated upward based on response of breakthrough pain. This dosing formulation has the advantage of a very rapid onset, generally 10 to 15 minutes.

Rectal—Rectal administration of opioids is useful in patients without IV access who cannot swallow or who have nausea or vomiting. Other potential advantages include partial avoidance of the "first pass effect," and no influence of upper GI motility or food on absorption. Both morphine and hydromorphone suppositories are commercially available, and morphine solution can be diluted in 10–20 mL of water and given as an enema. Both IR and SR morphine tablets can be given rectally with an effect equal to oral administration. Avoid rectal administration in neutropenic and thrombocytopenic patients, as well as in patients with diarrhea or fecal incontinence. We rarely treat patients chronically with rectal opioids. Rather, this route is useful for 1 or 2 doses of medication, until a more reliable route can be established for long-term use. It may prove useful as a temporary measure for a patient at home who loses intravenous access.

Intravenous infusion—This parenteral route is best for rapid dose titration. There are clinical circumstances where IV therapy is the best option: persistent nausea and vomiting, an inability to swallow, a risk of aspiration, and high dose therapy that would require taking too many tablets or placing too many patches.

The only side effect that is increased with IV therapy is sedation. Continuous IV infusion is preferred to intermittent IV bolus infusion, as there is less sedation from peak blood level effects, and less breakthrough pain as blood levels reach a trough. Any short-acting opioid agonist may be administered by IV infusion, including morphine, hydromorphone, and fentanyl. After adequate analgesia is obtained, patients may be converted to an equianalgesic oral or patch dose for chronic administration. IV infusion may actually be the preferred route in patients near the end of life, if rapid escalation of pain is expected.

Patient-controlled analgesia (PCA) pumps were first studied in the post-operative setting but have been found to be useful for chronic pain management as well. Patients who are alert and understand how to operate the pump are given control in titrating their dose, and they get more immediate relief of breakthrough pain. The same drugs used for IV infusion may be administered, and portable PCA pumps for ambulatory patients are also available. A PCA pump has four components: (1) a continuous infusion rate; (2) a breakthrough bolus dose that is usually equal to or one-half the continuous rate; (3) a breakthrough dose interval, which is usually 10, 15, or 20 minutes, and (4) a further restricting lock-out, which is usually not used (as it is not necessary) for palliative care patients.

Subcutaneous injection or infusion—The subcutaneous route is useful for patients without reliable IV access but who cannot take oral/transdermal medications. Subcutaneous doses are equal to IV doses, but the initial onset of action is generally similar to oral administration (15 to 30 minutes). Continuous subcutaneous infusions, with or without a PCA component, may be used for chronic pain. Both morphine and hydromorphone are well absorbed by this route, and the only limiting factor is volume. Generally a rate up to 10 mL/hr is well tolerated, and morphine and hydromorphone can be concentrated up to 25 mg/mL and 10 mg/mL, respectively.

Intrathecal or epidural infusion—Intrathecal and epidural catheters allow administration of opioids directly into the spinal column. These routes are useful for patients not responding to escalating doses of oral or parenteral opioids, for patients on very high doses of opioids, and for patients with intolerable adverse effects. The disadvantages of these catheters include cost, line occlusion or leaking, pump failure, and infection. We generally reserve use of intrathecal/epidural opioids in the palliative care setting when systemic opioid therapy has failed. Morphine, hydromorphone, and fentanyl may all be used safely.

Intramuscular injection—Intramuscular (IM) injection of opioids and other medicines should be avoided in palliative care. It is painful, inconvenient to administer, has unreliable absorption, and offers no advantage over either IV or subcutaneous injections.

Adverse effects

Opioids have well-characterized adverse effects, some of them severe, but most easily managed or prevented. Educating your patients on what to expect and anticipating adverse effects are keys to successful pain management with opioids.

Central nervous system effects—Sedation is the most common CNS effect of opioids, but tolerance tends to develop in 3 to 5 days. If sedation persists beyond that, try lowering the dose a bit. A low-dose stimulant such as methylphenidate may also be used. Patients who are sleep deprived due to uncontrolled pain may experience more sedation when opioids are initiated, and this should not be confused with respiratory depression.

Other less common CNS effects include hallucinations, nightmares, and myoclonus. Synthetic opioids (e.g., fentanyl or methadone) are less likely to cause hallucinations and nightmares.

Nausea/vomiting—Opioids stimulate the chemoreceptor trigger zone, cause increased vestibular sensitivity, and decrease GI motility. Soon after starting therapy these effects lead to nausea in more than 50% of patients. As with sedation, tolerance usually develops in 2 to 3 days, but some patients require an antiemetic.

Pruritus—All opioids (particularly morphine) cause histamine release from mast cells, which can lead to pruritus. Antihistamines such as diphenhydramine or hydroxyzine are usually only effective for mild pruritus, but they do cause additional sedation. Moderate to severe pruritus, while not life threatening, is very bothersome, and the best strategy in these patients is to change to a synthetic agent (e.g., fentanyl).

Constipation—This is an inevitable effect of all opioid agonists. Tolerance does not usually develop over time. The mechanisms of opioid-induced constipation include decreased intestinal peristalsis, decreased GI secretions, and delayed gastric emptying. Constipation increases as the opioid dose increases. All patients receiving chronic opioids should be placed on a bowel regimen before they develop constipation that includes a stimulant laxative, with the dose titrated to produce a bowel movement every 1 to 2 days. One-third of patients need suppositories or enemas in addition to oral laxatives.

Respiratory effects—Respiratory depression is the most feared acute adverse effect of opioids. The mechanism involves activation of opioid receptors in the brain stem, leading to decreased response of the respiratory center to carbon dioxide. It is unusual for this to be a problem for those with chronic or severe pain. Pain is a respiratory stimulant, and counteracts the effect of opioids. The dose of opioid is titrated until pain is relieved, achieving a "balanced" effect on the respiratory center. With higher dose therapy, sedation usually develops before respiratory depression. Note that with intrathecal/epidural administration, respiratory depression may be delayed up to 24 hours.

Cardiovascular effects—The most common cardiovascular effect of opioids is hypotension; histamine released from mast cells has a vasodilator effect. This is most common with morphine and is aggravated by hypovolemia. Bradycardia occurs less commonly.

Physical dependence—Physical dependence is a physiologic certainty with chronic opioid therapy. *It is completely distinct from psychological dependence.* Physical dependence simply means that abrupt discontinuation of the opioid or administration of an antagonist will result in withdrawal symptoms. These may include anxiety, irritability, chills, nausea/vomiting, diaphoresis, diarrhea, and abdominal cramps. Appropriately tapering the dose avoids these effects.

Psychological dependence—Also called "addiction," it is when a person seeks the drug for euphoria in the absence of pain. This is rarely observed in the palliative care patient population (less than 1%), but it is feared by patients and their families. Be sure to distinguish between true psychological addiction and "pseudo-addiction," which is a patient's demand for adequate analgesia to relieve pain that is misinterpreted by health care providers as drug-seeking behavior. The treatment for pseudo-addiction is pain relief.

Other Opioid-Like Agents

Non-opioid/opioid combinations

Available non-opioid/opioid combinations are listed in Table 2-4. These products usually contain acetaminophen plus codeine, hydrocodone, propoxyphene or oxycodone. Dose escalation is limited by the acetaminophen component, which should not exceed 4 grams per day chronically. These agents should be viewed as alternatives to non-opioids alone in mild to moderate pain and are actually best used for acute and temporary pain (i.e., after dental procedures or minor surgery). In palliative care, it is better to avoid combination products, and to titrate each of the analgesics individually.

Partial agonists (buprenorphine) and *agonists/antagonists* (butorphanol, nalbuphine, and pentazocine) all have a "soft ceiling" effect that limits our ability to escalate doses. They offer no advantage over pure opioid agonists and should be avoided in the palliative care patient.

Pure opioid antagonists

These include naloxone (IV only, Narcan) and naltrexone (oral only, Trexan). Naltrexone is used in detoxification programs to decrease cravings for opioids. Naloxone is almost exclusively used to reverse impending respiratory depression from opioids, usually following overdoses. Antagonists should be used cautiously in the palliative care patient on opioids for pain. These drugs not only reverse sedation and respiratory depression but also reverse all analgesia. Restrict your use of naloxone in palliative care to patients with profound respiratory depression (respiratory rate < 10/minute), who are not arousable, or when withdrawing opioids does not result in adequate restoration of breathing.

TABLE 2-4	*Non-Opioid/Opioid Combinations*

Trade Name	Drug Combination (per tablet)	Dosing
Darvocet N-50	Acetaminophen 325 mg Propoxyphene 50 mg	1–2 tabs PO Q4–6H
Darvocet N-100	Acetaminophen 325 mg Propoxyphene 100 mg	1–2 tabs PO Q4–6H
Lortab	Acetaminophen 500 mg Hydrocodone 2.5, 5, 7.5 mg	1–2 tabs PO Q4–6H
Lortab ES	Acetaminophen 650 mg Hydrocodone 10 mg	1 tab PO Q4–6H
Norco	Acetaminophen 325 mg Hydrocodone 10 mg	1–2 tabs PO Q4–6H
Percocet	Acetaminophen 325 or 650 mg Oxycodone 2.5, 5, 7.5, 10 mg	1–2 tabs PO Q4–6H
Percodan	Aspirin 325 mg Oxycodone 5 mg	1–2 tabs PO Q4–6H
Tylenol #3	Acetaminophen 300 mg Codeine 30 mg	1–2 tabs PO Q4–6H
Tylenol #4	Acetaminophen 300 mg Codeine 40 mg	1–2 tabs PO Q4–6H
Tylox	Acetaminophen 500 mg Oxycodone 5 mg	1–2 tabs PO Q4–6H
Vicodin	Acetaminophen 500 mg Hydrocodone 5 mg	1–2 tabs PO Q4–6H
Vicodin ES	Acetaminophen 750 mg Hydrocodone 7.5 mg	1 tab PO Q4–6H
Vicoprofen	Ibuprofen 200 mg Hydrocodone 7.5 mg	1–2 tabs PO Q4–6H

Note: Doses of acetaminophen should not exceed 4 grams/day.

Never give high dose naloxone by IV-push to an opioid tolerant patient: severe pain and symptoms of withdrawal will result. One amp (0.4 mg) of naloxone can be diluted in 10 mL normal saline and 0.5–1 mL given every few minutes. This allows gradual reversal of respiratory depression without completely reversing analgesia. Naloxone generally lasts 1 to 3 hours in patients with normal renal function; therefore, patients previously on SR tablets or patches may require re-dosing of naloxone.

Adjuvant Analgesics

There are a number of drug classes that have analgesic effects in certain circumstances (6). When combined with opioids they may provide better pain control with fewer side effects.

Antidepressants

Tricyclic antidepressants (TCAs) are useful as first-line adjuvant therapy for neuropathic pain syndromes. Unfortunately, many patients cannot tolerate the resultant sedation, or anti-cholinergic side effects like dry mouth, orthostasis, and constipation. This is especially true with geriatric patients. If used, amitriptyline or nortriptyline should be initiated at low doses (25 mg at bedtime, or 10 mg for elderly patients) and titrated upwards by 10–25 mg increments every few days as tolerated. Generally 100–150 mg is needed for analgesia. Remember to increase the dose appropriately; failure to titrate is the biggest mistake clinicians make in managing neuropathic pain. Onset of pain relief is delayed, generally occurring in 1 to 2 weeks, with maximum effects in 4 to 8 weeks.

Venlafaxine, an "atypical" antidepressant that inhibits reuptake of serotonin, norepinephrine, and dopamine, has shown promise in treating neuropathic pain and may be better tolerated than TCAs (7).

Anticonvulsants

Anticonvulsant drugs are also useful for neuropathic pain, as well as in treating myoclonus caused by high doses of opioids. Clinical experience is greatest with carbamazepine. Initiate therapy at 100 mg three times daily (or once daily for elderly patients), and titrate the dose to a therapeutic plasma level (4–12 mcg/mL). Agranulocytosis is the greatest concern with carbamazepine, and monitoring blood counts is necessary. Patients with bone marrow compromise should be considered for an alternative anticonvulsant, such as phenytoin, valproic acid, clonazepam, or phenytoin.

Gabapentin is a relatively new anticonvulsant for treatment of pain, and has a good adverse effect profile and no significant drug interactions (8). Initiate therapy at low doses (100 mg three times daily), and increase every few days to target 900 mg per day. Some patients may require up to 3600 mg per day.

Corticosteroids

Indications for adjuvant corticosteroid therapy are numerous and include refractory neuropathic pain, bone pain, visceral obstructive pain, pain caused by lymphedema, headache from increased intracranial pressure, back pain due to spinal cord compression, and pain from soft tissue infiltration by tumor. The analgesic effects of corticosteroids are related to their ability to reduce capillary permeability and the mass effect of edema, as well as their anti-inflammatory effects. Mood elevation as well as depression may be an indirect effect.

We usually start with dexamethasone, 4 mg two to four times daily. Prednisone is a reasonable alternative at equipotent doses (20–30 mg). You may attempt a taper after initial dosing to minimize adverse effects, but some patients will require continued therapy for maximal pain control.

The benefits of steroids tend to outweigh adverse effects in the palliative care setting, even though potential adverse effects are numerous. These include myopathy, opportunistic infections, gastritis and ulcers, exacerbation of diabetes, peripheral edema, hypokalemia, osteoporosis, and hypertension. Acute psychiatric complications, including mania and frank psychosis, may occur within the first few weeks of therapy and respond promptly to dose reduction or discontinuation.

Bisphosphonates

The indication for therapy is bone pain caused by metastatic cancer. Pamidronate was first approved to treat the hypercalcemia of malignancy. As adjunctive therapy, it reduces opioid analgesic use, a need for radiation therapy to control pain, and the risk of pathological fracture. The mechanism is thought to involve inhibition of cancer-related, osteoclast-induced bone resorption. The recommended dose of pamidronate is 90 mg IV over 2 hours, given every 3 to 4 weeks. Zolendronic acid (Zometa) may also be used at doses of 4 mg IV over 15 minutes. Oral bisphosphonates (e.g., alendronate) should be avoided in the palliative care patient due to variable bioavailability and the high incidence of GI adverse effects.

Ketamine

In addition to being an anesthetic, ketamine is an N-methyl-d-aspartate (NMDA) antagonist (9). The excitatory amino acid glutamate acts at the NMDA receptor. Animal models have shown that activation of NMDA decreases the magnitude and duration of opioid-induced analgesia. NMDA antagonists increase opioid sensitivity.

In sub-anesthestic doses ketmine (0.1 mg/kg vs. 1 mg/kg used as anesthesia) decreases opioid requirements and allows rapid control of pain in previously refractory patients. It is a drug not commonly needed, but it is good to keep in mind for patients who have continued severe pain despite aggressive opioid dose escalation.

Other Symptoms

Nausea and Vomiting

Two-thirds of palliative care patients will experience nausea and/or vomiting (10). Vomiting tends to be more responsive to drug therapy than nausea.

The differential diagnosis of nausea/vomiting in the palliative care patient is long but can broadly be classified into the following: (1) *Gastrointestinal*, including bowel obstruction, hepatomegaly, constipation, ascites, and peptic ulcer disease, or gastritis; (2) *Neurologic*, including increased intracranial pressure, severe or chronic pain, and anxiety; (3) *Metabolic*, including hypercalcemia, hyponatremia, uremia, and hypoadrenalism; and (4) *Medication-related*, including anti-neoplastics, opioids, digitalis glycosides, iron supplements, NSAIDs, and anesthetics.

Whenever possible, treat the underlying cause of nausea/vomiting, and use antiemetics for refractory symptoms (Table 2-5) (10).

Dopamine antagonists—They block dopamine receptors in the chemoreceptor trigger zone in the CNS. Adverse effects include sedation, hypotension, anticholinergic effects, and extrapyramidal symptoms (dystonia and akathesia). Metoclopramide also causes diarrhea by increasing GI motility. All phenothiazines and butyrophenones may prolong the QT interval, provoking ventricular arrhythmias. Droperidol is especially arrhythmogenic.

The dopamine antagonists (i.e., haloperidol) are useful as first-line agents for most types of end-of-life nausea/vomiting. They

TABLE 2-5	*Antiemetic Drugs*		

Generic Name	Trade Name	Dosing	Role in Palliative Care
Dopamine Antagonists			
Droperidol	Inapsine	IV: 2.5–5 mg Q3–4H	1st line for most
Haloperidol	Haldol	IV & PO: 1–2 mg Q6–8H	patients; *avoid*
Metoclopramide	Reglan	IV & PO: 10–20 mg Q6H	promethazine
Prochlorperazine	Compazine	IV & PO: 10 mg Q4–6H PR: 25 mg Q6H	due to sedation.
Promethazine	Phenergan	IV/PO/PR: 12.5–25 mg Q6–8H IV/PO/PR: 10 mg Q6–8H	
Thiethylperazine	Torecan		
Serotonin Antagonists			
Dolasetron	Anzemet	IV & PO: 100 mg Q24H	2nd or 3rd line for
Granisetron	Kytril	IV: 1 mg Q24H PO: 1–2 mg Q24H	most patients; 1st line in AMS.
Ondansetron	Zofran	IV: 4–8 mg Q8–24H PO: 8 mg Q8–12H	
Benzodiazepines			
Diazepam	Valium	IV & PO: 2–10 mg Q6–12H	1st line for patients
Lorazepam	Ativan	IV & PO: 1–2 mg Q6–8H	with anxiety; 2nd line in others.
Corticosteroids			
Dexamethasone	Decadron	IV & PO: 2–4 mg Q6–12H	2nd line.
Cannabinoids			
Dronabinol	Marinol	PO: 2.5–10 mg Q6–12H	3rd line.
Octreotide	Sandostatin	SC: 50–100 mcg SC Q8H	1st line for bowel obstruction.

IV = intravenous; PO = oral; SC = subcutaneous; AMS = altered mental status.

have the added advantage of being available in the most flexible dosage forms (tablets, injectables, suppositories). Avoid the use of promethazine if at all possible due to excessive sedation with this agent. Due to pro-motility effects, metoclopramide is particularly useful for GI-related nausea.

Serotonin antagonists—Marketed primarily for chemotherapy-induced and post-operative nausea and vomiting, they act by selectively blocking the serotonin type-3 receptor located on vagal afferent neurons in the GI tract. They are quite well tolerated (side effects include headache, constipation, and occasional increases in serum liver transaminases). On the other hand, serotonin blockers are no more effective than other drug classes, and they are expensive. We use them when other classes of antiemetics do not work. One exception: they have by far the fewest CNS effects and may be used first-line in patients with altered mental status. All are available as injectables and tablets, and ondansetron is also formulated as an oral disintegrating tablet for patients who cannot swallow.

Benzodiazepines—This drug class activates the γ-aminobutyric acid (GABA) receptor, leading to antiemetic, amnestic, and anxiolytic effects. They are most effective in patients with anxiety associated with their nausea. Any benzodiazepine can be used, although diazepam (long acting) and lorazepam (short acting) are the most widely studied and readily available. Adverse effects include sedation, disinhibition, hallucinations, motor incoordination, and occasionally, paradoxical CNS excitation in children and the elderly. Diazepam and lorazepam are available for both oral and parenteral administration, and lorazepam gels are effective when applied topically. You may have good results with lorazepam tablets sublingually when a patient cannot swallow.

Corticosteroids—Dexamethasone and prednisone are the corticosteroids most widely used as antiemetics. Their mechanism of action is not clear but may involve decreased serotonin turnover in the CNS and modulation of higher cortical pathways that activate the vomiting center. Adverse effects can be limiting and include euphoria, insomnia, hyperglycemia, hypertension, and immunosuppression with long-term use. In palliative care, I find corticosteroids to be most useful in pain management, but they are useful as second-line agents for nausea/vomiting.

Cannabinoids—The only cannabinoid available as a drug is dronabinol, an oral capsule (11). Cannabinoids likely act as antiemetics by depressing higher cortical pathways that activate the emetic center. Adverse effects can be bothersome to patients, particularly those who have not used cannabinoids recreationally. These effects include sedation, euphoria, dysphoria, halluci-nations, memory loss, and motor incoordination. Patients often report to me that dronabinol makes them "think funny," and find it an unpleasant experience.

A discussion of the merits of "medical marijuana" are beyond the scope of this chapter, but patients who claim that smoking marijuana is more effective than the capsules may be correct (11). Inhaled forms do not undergo a first-pass effect and attain higher peak concentrations. Cannabinoids may be better appetite stimulants than antiemetics, and most reserve them for third-line use for control of nausea/vomiting.

Octreotide—There is a niche for octreotide as an antiemetic (10). It globally decreases GI secretions and is the best drug to use for nausea associated with *bowel obstruction*. This type of nausea is generally refractory to all other antiemetics, and octreotide can provide significant relief with minimal adverse effects. The most limiting issue is that it must be given as a subcutaneous injection three times daily. A monthly intramuscular depot formulation is available; however, in palliative care patients, the delayed onset makes this formulation impractical.

Anorexia and Cachexia

Anorexia (decreased appetite) is experienced by 85% of patients near the end of life. Cachexia includes marked weight loss with muscle wasting and is due to increased metabolic rate with elevated cytokine production. It is best described in the cancer population but is seen with other chronic illnesses including end-stage heart, liver, kidney, and lung disease.

Anorexia may occur with numerous disorders, including gastrointestinal obstruction, dehydration, constipation, nausea/vomiting, pain, fatigue, depression, and other disease states, such as liver and renal disease, advanced heart failure, and malignancy. Treating an underlying process will help, and there are several medications that can help by stimulating appetite.

Perhaps the least expensive is methyphenidate (Ritalin). This nonspecific central nervous system stimulant is not approved for this purpose, but it works as an appetite stimulant for many patients. Start at 10 mg three times a day; if it works it does so within a few days. If not, try one of the following.

Megestrol acetate—Megestrol is a synthetic progestin still used as a treatment for hormone-responsive breast and prostate cancers. It is first-line therapy for appetite stimulation in palliative care.

Doses for this indication are much higher than anti-cancer doses, generally 400–800 mg daily. Because the largest tablet size is 40 mg, use the oral suspension (40 mg/mL). It is less expensive and more convenient than pills. The primary adverse effects of megestrol include edema and a small risk of thrombotic events. Give patients a several week drug trial before calling megestrol a therapeutic failure.

Cannabinoids—As mentioned above, many patients find dronabinol an unpleasant drug to take. If the patient is willing, it is a reasonable second-line appetite stimulant. Start at low doses (2.5 mg two to four times daily) to minimize CNS adverse effects, and titrate up to a maximum of 10 mg four times a day.

Corticosteroids—Steroids may be considered for patients with refractory anorexia. Doses needed for this indication are much smaller than those used for pain or nausea: dexamethasone 2–4 mg or prednisone 15–20 mg daily. These drugs are much less expensive than megestrol and dronabinol and may also be given parenterally.

Constipation and Bowel Obstruction

Constipation occurs in as many as two-thirds of palliative care patients. The etiology is often multifactorial. For most patients inactivity has a role, and dehydration and inadequate nutrition also contribute. Do not overlook metabolic abnormalities such as hypercalcemia, hypokalemia, and hypothyroidism. In the palliative setting, mechanical bowel obstruction can result from fecal impaction as well as intrabdominal tumor.

Perhaps the most common cause of constipation in the palliative setting is *drug therapy*, with opioids the usual etiology. Other drug causes of constipation include vinca alkaloid chemotherapy, serotonin antagonist antiemetics, iron supplements, aluminum and calcium-containing antacids, anticholinergics, calcium channel blockers, and Carafate. When drug therapy is responsible, stopping the offending drug is desirable but not always possible. Patients needing opioids for pain control must continue them, and laxative therapy is needed. In fact, those starting opioid therapy should also begin laxative therapy as prophylaxis.

Laxatives—Laxatives that are commonly used are listed in Table 2-6. There are a few general principles of laxative use. First, emollient laxatives, also called stool softeners, do nothing to

TABLE 2-6	Laxatives for Management of Constipation	

Laxative Class	Dosing	Pharmacology
Emollient Laxatives Docusate Ca (Surfak) Docusate Na (Colace)	 50–100 mg PO QD–QID 50–100 mg PO QD–QID	Surfactants that promote water and electrolyte secretion; also termed "stool softeners."
Lubricant Laxatives Mineral oil Glycerin	 15–60 mL PO QD Suppository PR QD–BID	Lubricate stool surface.
Saline Laxatives Magnesium citrate Magnesium hydroxide sodium phosphates (Fleets)	 1/2–1 bottle PO ×1 30–60 mL PO QD–BID PO: 20–30 mL PO ×1 PR: enema ×1	Cations and anions that cause an osmotic effect, increasing intraluminal water content; also cause release of cholecystokinin, which stimulates intestinal motility.
Stimulant Laxatives Bisacodyl (Dulcolax) Casanthranol + docusate (Peri-Colace) Castor oil Senna ± docusate (Senoakot)	 PO: 5–15 mg QD–TID PR: 10 mg QD 1–2 tabs PO QD–TID 15–60 mL PO ×1 1–3 tabs PO QD–TID	Direct stimulation of the mysenteric plexus, which causes increased peristalsis in the distal ileum and colon.
Hyperosmotic Laxatives Lactulose Sorbitol	 15–60 mL PO QD–BID 30 mL PO QD–BID	Osmotic agents of nonabsorbed sugars that increase water secretion into the GI lumen.

stimulate the GI tract to move. Use them with a stimulant or other laxative. Second, oral administration is preferred for chronic treatment and prevention of constipation. Reserve rectal suppositories and enemas for refractory patients and one-time use. Third, when patients have constipation caused by drugs that inhibit GI motility (e.g., opioids), chronic use of stimulant laxatives is the standard of care and will not cause "laxative abuse" in patients. Finally, before using aggressive oral laxatives to correct constipation, rule-out fecal impaction first. This condition will require therapy with enemas prior to initiating oral therapies.

Octreotide—As discussed above octreotide is one of the best supportive drugs for the management of bowel obstruction. The immediate-release form is most often used (rather than the monthly depot) and doses should start at 50 mcg subcutaneous (SC) three times daily. Titrate upward every few days by 50 mcg increments until symptomatic relief is achieved. Most palliative care patients respond at doses of 200 mcg or less, but doses up to 500 mcg SC three times daily are safe and well tolerated. The most common adverse effects of octreotide include diarrhea, flushing, and hypoglycemia.

Delirium

Acute confusional states occur in more than half of those near the end of life (12). The distressing symptoms may include altered consciousness, decreased comprehension, restlessness, and hallucinations. The etiology is often multifactorial, and can include infection, metabolic disorders like hypoxemia, dehydration, hyponatremia, hypercalcemia, uremia, and hepatic encephalopathy. When the nurse calls you late at night about new mental status changes, check a finger-tip oxygen saturation. Withdrawal from medicines may be responsible (opioids, benzodiazepines, psychotropics, alcohol). Underlying psychiatric conditions such as severe anxiety make delirium more common in the palliative setting. Elderly patients in hospital are subject to "sun-downing." Those with mild cognitive impairment are especially prone to this. When a precipitating factor cannot be identified or eliminated, antipsychotic therapy is needed.

Antipsychotics—Haloperidol is the most often used and effective drug for treatment of delirium in the dying patient (12). Relatively low dose therapy works, generally 1–2 mg every 6 to 12 hours. Oral use is effective if the patient is able to swallow, and IV administration works promptly. Intramuscular injections are also effective, but absorption may be erratic. Monitor carefully for acute dystonic reactions, particularly in younger patients. These may be treated with lorazepam, diphenhydramine, or benztropine. Long-term effects of haloperidol, such as tardive dyskinesia, are generally not a concern in the palliative care setting. More recently, atypical antipsychotics have been used to treat delirium. Risperidone is a good second-line agent at doses starting at 0.5 mg twice daily.

Anxiolytics—Benzodiazepines may be used as well, and in combination with haloperidol. Avoid the use of slow-onset agents such as diazepam if immediate effects are desired. Lorazepam is more useful with its rapid onset. Lorazepam also has the advantage of being effective orally, sublingually, parenterally, and when administered topically as a gel. A starting dose is 1–2 mg, which can be increased and then given as often as every 4 hours. Elderly and cachectic patients may have dramatic responses with much lower doses: start with 0.5 mg.

Dyspnea

There are many possible causes of "air hunger" in dying patients: obstructive lung disease, pneumonia, progression of lung cancer, heart failure, pleural effusion, pulmonary embolus, abdominal distension (ascites, bowel obstruction), and others. When the underlying cause cannot be fully relieved, other medications may be added. Supplemental oxygen and bronchodilators may lead to symptomatic improvement, even if oxygen saturation is in the normal range.

Opioids—Using morphine to treat dyspnea takes advantage of one of its most feared adverse effects, respiratory depression. Morphine decreases the brain stem response to rising carbon dioxide levels, decreases the respiratory drive, and leads patients to feel like they are no longer "gasping for air." Low dose morphine usually works, often 1 mg/hr as a continuous infusion or 5–10 mg oral doses. The nature of this symptom calls for rapid relief. Sublingual morphine is rapidly absorbed, using either oral morphine tablets or concentrated solutions placed under the tongue. The parenteral routes are also effective. Most recently, there have been reports of inhaled morphine at doses of 20 mg by hand-held nebulizer leading to rapid reversal of dyspnea. Morphine is by far the most commonly used opioid for this purpose, but other opioids would be effective as well.

Anticholinergics—Excessive bronchial secretions often accompany dyspnea in the dying patient. For those able to swallow pills, try glycopyrrolate (Robinul), 1–2 mg at 8- to 12-hour intervals. If unable to swallow, the transdermal scopolamine patch is a good alternative (1 or 2 patches behind the ear, changed every 3 days).

References

1. Brant JM. The art of palliative care: living with hope, dying with dignity. Oncol Nurs Forum 1998;25:995–1004.

2. Levy MH. Pain management in advanced cancer. Semin Oncol 1985;12:394–410.

3. Eisenberg E, Berkey CS, Carr DB, et al. Efficacy and safety of nonsteroidal anti-inflammatory drugs for cancer pain: a meta-analysis. J Clin Oncol 1994;12:2756–2765.

4. Cherny NI. Opioid analgesics: comparative features and prescribing guidelines. Drugs 1996;51:713–737.

5. Agency for Health Care Policy and Research. Clinical practice guideline: management of cancer pain. Rockville, Maryland: AHCPR Publication No. 94-0592, 1994.

6. Portenoy RK. Adjuvant analgesic agents. Hematol Oncol Clinics North Am 1996;10:103–119.

7. Sumpton JE, Moulin DE. Treatment of neuropathic pain with venlafaxine. Ann Pharmacother 2001;35:557–559.

8. Laird MA, Gidal BE. Use of gabapentin in the treatment of neuropathic pain. Ann Pharmacother 2000;34:802–807.

9. Fine PG. Low-dose ketamine in the management of opioid nonresponsive terminal cancer pain. J Pain Symptom Manage 1999;17:296–300.

10. Mitchelson F. Pharmacological agents affecting emesis: A review (parts I and II). Drugs 1992;43:295–315 & 443–463.

11. Williamson EM, Evans FJ. Cannabinoids in clinical practice. Drugs 2000;60:1303–1314.

12. Casarett DJ, Inouye SK. Diagnosis and management of delirium near the end of life. Ann Intern Med 2001;135:32–40.

3 Heart Disease

George J. Taylor

Congestive Heart Failure

Epidemiology, Natural History, Prognosis, and Clinical Decisions

Congestive heart failure (CHF) is the clinical syndrome caused by insufficient cardiac output, leading to either pulmonary or systemic congestion. About 400,000 new patients are diagnosed annually in the United States, and almost 3 million patients have CHF. It is the most common admitting diagnoses for old people, and the incidence of CHF more than doubles with each decade over age 45. We may expect reduced mortality in middle age from coronary artery disease, resulting in an even larger elderly population at risk for CHF.

Some patients with CHF have extracardiac or valvular heart disease that limits cardiac output, even though ventricular function is normal. Surgical correction of the underlying process may offer a cure. However, most of the patients we encounter with end-stage CHF have left ventricular (LV) dysfunction. The most common etiology is coronary artery disease, followed by hypertensive heart disease and idiopathic, dilated cardiomyopathy.

Increased myocardial stiffness prevents LV filling during diastole and limits stroke volume and cardiac output. Patients with CHF and "diastolic dysfunction," by definition, have normal left ventricular ejection fraction (LVEF). When compared with CHF caused by systolic dysfunction (low LVEF), the prognosis with diastolic heart failure is better, and symptoms are more easily controlled. Diastolic dysfunction accounts for a small minority of those with end-stage CHF.

Prognosis

The early clinical trials of angiotensin converting enzyme (ACE) inhibitor therapy included placebo groups (Table 3-1) (1). Patients receiving placebo also were treated with diuretics and digoxin. Their 1-year mortality with New York Heart Association (NYHA)

TABLE 3-1	*Indicators of Poor Prognosis with Congestive Heart Failure*

A. Functional Class

*NYHA Class**	*1-Year Mortality***
I	5–10%
II–III	15–30%
IV	50–60%

B. Other indicators of bad prognosis***

Clinical
    Coronary artery disease etiology
    Resting tachycardia
    Low blood pressure
    Narrow pulse pressure
    S_3 gallop
    Cardiac cachexia
    Male sex

Hemodynamic
    Low LV ejection fraction
    Elevated LV end-diastolic pressure
    Low cardiac output

Clinical laboratory
    Low serum sodium
    Elevated plasma renin activity and aldosterone
    Elevated atrial and brain natriuretic peptide
    Low potassium, magnesium

Cardiac rhythm
    Sinus tachycardia
    Atrial fibrillation
    Frequent ventricular ectopics
    Ventricular tachycardia

---

* New York Heart Association (NYHA) functional class: I, asymptomatic with low left ventricular (LV) ejection fraction; II, symptoms with vigorous activity (able to walk 3 blocks); III, symptoms with mild exertion; IV, symptoms at rest.
** Estimates of mortality are based upon a number of recent clinical trials (1).
*** Thus, a patient with moderate symptoms (NYHA II–III) who also has resting tachycardia, low blood pressure, a gallop, and low serum sodium has an estimated 1-year mortality closer to 30%.

Class IV symptoms was 50% to 60%, and with Class II–III symptoms, 15% to 30%. Asymptomatic patients with poor LV function (Class I) had 5% to 10% 1-year mortality.

There are a number of markers of poor prognosis with CHF (Table 3-1). They are usually found in combination. The patient with poor exercise tolerance, resting tachycardia (a particularly ominous finding), and an S_3 gallop usually has low LVEF and a thin walled LV. Poor prognosis is confirmed by low serum sodium which is a marker of elevated plasma renin activity. When such a patient requires frequent hospitalization for control of congestion, or when diuresis is complicated by hypotension, you may correctly infer that the patient is "end-stage." Even with optimal modern therapy using ACE inhibitors and beta blockers, the annual death rate remains high (2).

Tough Decisions for the End-Stage Patient: Palliative Care Versus Possible Life-Saving Procedures

The drug therapies that prolong survival also control symptoms and thus are an element of palliative care. A dilemma in cardiovascular medicine is that many of our treatments are mechanical. At end of life, it seems that there is often an interventional or surgical procedure that is possible, a possibility that represents a tough choice for the patient and doctor.

Erring on the side of aggressive, interventional therapy may remove any chance for a peaceful death. You may be telling your patient, "You can die soon with CHF or sudden death, or you can die after a couple weeks in the intensive care unit with ventilator, incision, and chest tube. Or maybe you survive the surgery, but it does not improve the quality of your life. We all may feel that you have suffered in vain."

Erring the other way may cheat the patient of months, perhaps years of useful life. The patient gets a different message: "You can die now, or take a chance, struggle through an operation, and live fairly well for some time."

Patients—and their doctors—tend to believe that mechanical/surgical treatments are "curative" and "work," while medical therapy is "palliative" and therefore less effective. Of course, that is not how life works. The effectiveness of any treatment is based largely on patient selection, whether surgical or medical. Clinical judgment is the process of sensibly matching the patient and therapy.

Considering surgery for advanced *valvular* heart disease

Aortic stenosis—There are a couple of situations where surgery for valvular heart disease may be useful, even with advanced symptoms. That may be the case with aortic stenosis (AS). The tight aortic valve increases LV afterload, and replacing it is afterload reduction therapy. Left ventricular ejection fraction improves with dramatic improvement in symptoms. Prognosis after surgery is quite good, and aortic valve replacement can be recommended for otherwise healthy octogenarians.

Mitral stenosis—This may cause occult heart failure in elderly patients, usually women. With low cardiac output and flow across the valve the murmur may be soft or inaudible. Often the diagnosis is an incidental finding on chest x-ray or echocardiogram; excluding occult valvular disease is one argument for a screening echocardiogram for those with CHF. Most patients with mitral stenosis (MS) have normal left ventricular function, and thus have a good prognosis with valve replacement.

Mitral regurgitation—Mitral regurgitation (MR) may not be amenable to surgical repair once symptoms are advanced (3). The problem is the effect of MR on LV afterload and function. Think of afterload as the impedance to LV ejection. With normal valves, impedance is a function of vascular resistance and blood pressure. A stenotic aortic valve impedes LV emptying, and replacement of the valve "uncorks" the ventricle.

Mitral regurgitation is different. Since the LV empties into both the left atrium (LA) and aorta, impedance to LV ejection is a mixture of LA and aortic pressure. Left atrial pressure is low, about 15 mm Hg, so net afterload is low. Replacing the leaking valve removes the LA as a low pressure dump for LV ejection. Left ventricular afterload is higher after surgery, and LV function thus worsens.

You may thus expect LVEF to worsen after mitral valve replacement for MR. Preserving papillary muscle function helps overall LV performance, making valve repair superior to replacement when function is borderline. Even with repair, the patient with reduced LVEF or with a dilated LV that fails to contract to nearly normal size with systole has high surgical mortality. Those who survive the operation are often left with the symptoms and prognosis of advanced cardiomyopathy. In general, surgery is not recommended for MR when LVEF is below 40% or the LV end-systolic dimension exceeds 5.5 cm on the echocardiogram.

Mitral regurgitation may be a complication of CHF rather than the cause. LV dilation alters the geometry of the papillary muscle and (perhaps) stretches the mitral ring leading to regurgitation. That is usually the case with the patient who has dilated cardiomyopathy, a soft murmur and an echo report stating "moderate MR." Repairing the valve does nothing for symptoms or prognosis.

Aortic regurgitation—Aortic regurgitation (AR) is a volume overload condition like MR. But with AR there is also an increase in LV afterload, and patients have an increase in LV thickness as well as chamber size. Like MR, ejection fraction and LV end-systolic dimension are guides to the risk of surgery. When these measures are unfavorable, successful valve replacement may leave the patient with persistent CHF. (Since afterload is elevated, vasodilator therapy is more successful for AR than it is for MR.)

Considering revascularization for ischemic cardiomyopathy

This clinical dilemma typically involves a patient with coronary disease who has had multiple operations or interventional procedures. Symptoms may be anginal or congestive. A successful procedure requires a coronary artery that is large enough and disease-free so that bypass or angioplasty can work (a "good target").

The artery must also supply viable muscle, as restoring blood flow to scar does no good. At times there is uncertainty about viability, as live but chronically ischemic muscle may have little contractility. A nuclear "viability study" (a variation on the thallium perfusion scan) may help identify hibernating muscle.

Low LVEF, alone, is not a contraindication to revascularization, though it indicates increased risk. Another reliable guide is symptoms. Patients with low LVEF but good exercise tolerance and mild or no congestion do well with surgery. Those with class III–IV heart failure do poorly.

Coronary artery surgery, as a rule, is not a reliable therapy for those who have CHF but no apparent ischemia. When there is angina plus CHF, bypass surgery may be an alternative to cardiac transplantation.

Angioplasty and stenting are less invasive than coronary bypass surgery, with far less morbidity. A rationale for angiography in the end-stage patient is the hope of finding a symptom-causing lesion that can be palliated using a catheter-based technique. In practice, this is frequently the case for the elderly patient with no prior history of coronary artery disease. It is less common to find a "culprit lesion" that can be dilated in the patient who has a long history of coronary artery disease (CAD) and multiple revascularization procedures.

"Redo" bypass surgery is even a higher risk with advanced age. A colleague with insight pointed out that for a person who has lived to the late 70s or into the 80s, longevity is less important than other considerations (Chapter 1). In most cases it is the patient who makes the decision to avoid more procedures. When the patient with a history of multiple vascular procedures states, "I've had enough," the seasoned clinician accepts this decision, and shifts to the palliative mode.

Ventricular arrhythmias

Sudden death is common in patients with reduced LVEF, and the usual mechanism is ventricular fibrillation. Ambulatory monitoring studies after myocardial infarction found that complex ventricular arrhythmias (VA) and low LVEF go hand-in-hand. Those with low LVEF who have symptomatic VAs or ventricular tachycardia (VT) that can be provoked during electrophysiology study are high risk for sudden death.

The Cardiac Arrhythmia Suppression Trial (CAST) found that suppression of the arrhythmias with drug therapy is of no use (4). In fact, the proarrhythmic effect of membrane active antiarrhythmic agents outweighs benefits. With therapy the ambulatory monitor looked better, but the rate of sudden death was higher. There are situations where drug therapy helps: (1) although beta blockade does not suppress VAs on the ambulatory monitor, it does lower the risk of sudden death, (2) amiodarone may be used to suppress symptomatic VAs in patients with reduced LVEF with relative safety.

The most effective treatment for the prevention of sudden cardiac death is the implantable cardioverter defibrillator (ICD). Its efficacy has been proven in clinical trials, and in practice it is unusual to have a patient die suddenly who has a functioning ICD.

In individual cases, argument can be made against ICD therapy: (1) Discharge of the ICD hurts. An occasional patient develops excessive anxiety in anticipation of being shocked, and ICDs have been taken out for this reason. (2) Sudden cardiac death is a relatively peaceful death, and the ICD removes this possibility. The patient with CHF and advanced symptoms may prefer this to an alternative that is more uncomfortable (i.e., pulmonary edema), or prolonged (i.e., a low output state with congestion alternating with shock). For a given patient, this would be a rational decision that is not far from what we do in daily practice. We typically avoid electrophysiology study when dealing with advanced CHF, even though we know that VT is ubiquitous. If we studied all end-stage patients we would find plenty who have inducible VT, but we reserve study for those with symptomatic arrhythmias who do not appear to be at end of life. (3) ICD therapy is expensive, an issue for many patients when they are weighing benefits against all costs (financial and personal, Chapter 1).

New interventional therapies for left ventricular dysfunction

A number of techniques are being tested in clinical trials for their effects on symptoms and survival. Resection of a portion of the LV to reduce LV size may improve performance, as LV wall tension is proportional to radius of the chamber (the Laplace relationship). Wall tension is proportional to myocardial oxygen demand.

A new pacing technology has been developed that allows pacing the LV from two different LV sites, so-called "resynchronization" therapy (5). It is used for patients with cardiomyopathy and left bundle branch block. This conduction abnormality causes late activation of the interventricular septum, reducing LV stroke volume and cardiac output. Simultaneous pacing of both the LV septum and lateral wall allows them to contract together, improving stroke volume without increasing myocardial work or oxygen requirement. Early trials have found improved exercise tolerance, functional class, and quality of life. It is still new and it will be an expensive technology.

Heart transplantation

Transplantation relieves symptoms and prolongs survival for the end-stage patients. Indications and contraindications are summarized in Box 3-1; most heart failure patients are not candidates. There is a shortage of organs, and it is estimated that fewer than 20% of those who are candidates for transplant get it. While transplantation and artificial heart technology are interesting to follow, they are the sideshow, and the big tent is still medical therapy for the large population of people with heart failure.

> ### BOX 3-1 | *Heart transplantation*
>
> **Indications**
> End-stage congestive heart failure
>   Cardiogenic shock requiring mechanical assistance
>   Low output state requiring continuous intravenous inotropic
>   support
>   NYHA class III or IV CHF and poor 12-month survival (Table 3-1)
> Refractory angina pectoris, unsuitable for revascularization
>   Symptoms prevent normal daily activities
>   Objective evidence for ischemia
>   Recurrent hospitalization for unstable angina
>   Life-threatening coronary anatomy
> Hypertrophic cardiomyopathy and NYHA class IV symptoms (Table
>   3-1)
> Life-threatening ventricular arrhythmia that cannot be controlled
>
> **Contraindications**
> Advanced age (varies, but some programs transplant into the 60s)
> Irreversible lung, kidney, or liver disease
> Diabetes plus end-organ disease
> Active infection
> Cancer
> Poor medical compliance
> Pulmonary hypertension (severe)
> Systemic disease limiting survival or rehabilitation
> Inadequate social support*
>
> ---
>
> * A nebulous category. Programs are reluctant to transplant a patient who does
> not have adequate family support. A "team" is needed to get a person through
> this complicated and difficult treatment, and equally difficult follow-up.
> "Support" includes financial resources. Though partially funded by the state,
> transplantation and follow-up are expensive, and no program can afford to give
> it away.

What to Tell the Patient with CHF

The medicines that are used to prolong survival also relieve
congestion, and all are appropriately recommended for the patient
with end-stage disease. That influences what we are able to tell our
patients. It is important to be honest about prognosis, and some
patients want to know their odds of dying (Table 3-1). But I am

| BOX 3-2 | *A doctor discusses the risk of dying with heart failure* |

"Any heart disease can be fatal, and I am sure that comes as no surprise to you. In your case, this is not predictable, and it may be misleading to talk about 'how much time you have.' In that regard, heart failure is different than many other serious illnesses. For example, most people with advanced lung cancer are gone in 6 to 12 months. But that is not true of heart disease (either CHF or CAD). Many people with heart disease like yours get better with treatment and live for years. For this reason, while your illness could be fatal, it is also true that you and I could be visiting in this clinic 5 or 10 or 20 years from now.

"How should you feel? It is normal to become depressed when hearing that you have heart disease. My experience is that most people feel better when they realize they have a chance of doing well. And they feel better yet as time goes by and they realize that their symptoms are improving with effective treatment. Eventually, most people take each day as it comes, and enjoy life."

quick to point out that the published risks may not be as applicable to the individual patient with heart disease as they are with some other illnesses. Box 3-2 is a sample of a typical conversation.

Obviously, a conversation like this with a patient must be adapted to your personality and the patient's. It usually takes place in stages over multiple office visits, and includes answering the patient's questions. (These sample dialogues are not scripts to be memorized and blurted out after taking a deep breath!) It may help to begin the discussion with questions: What have you heard about heart failure, and what does it mean to you? Has there been anyone in your family with heart failure, and how did they do? What scares you most about this illness?

At some point in your discussions, it may help to describe the control of advanced symptoms, especially dyspnea. A patient may be concerned about being on a ventilator. Point out that there are effective medical therapies for worsening dyspnea, and that ventilator therapy can be avoided. This would be a good time for the patient, family and you to decide on limits of care, and to be sure that advance directives are in place (Chapter 1).

One thing I would encourage you *not* to say is "there is nothing we can do for you." (How many times have patients told you they have heard that from doctors?) In the first place it is untrue. The medical treatment of end-stage CHF can be remarkably effective, and you should emphasize this. We may not have a "cure," a treatment that restores LV function to normal. But we do not have "cures" for many other chronic illnesses (diabetes comes to mind), and yet continue to offer hope. It is not false hope.

Finally, at some point mention practical, family matters such as having a will, life insurance, and other business affairs in order. This is not the first item on the agenda, but I consider it a part of my responsibility to any seriously ill patient. It is common for family members to ask the doctor to bring this up.

Palliative Treatment for End-Stage Congestive Heart Failure

Hospice care

A person with end-stage CHF who is frequently admitted to the hospital for diuresis and has declining quality of life may reasonably elect to avoid aggressive treatment, including cardiopulmonary resuscitation. At this stage of the illness it is helpful to enroll the patient in a hospice program. The hospice nurse and team make a big difference: intravenous medicines can be given at home and there is more effective regulation of dietary sodium and fluid intake. Any increase in congestion is detected early and is easier to correct, thus avoiding hospitalization. I am struck by how often symptoms resolve and exercise tolerance improves when regular hospice visits begin.

Drug therapy

When discussing treatment of CHF emphasis is usually on the effect of a drug on survival. Many of the following therapies have been shown to reduce mortality. Invariably, they also relieve symptoms, increase exercise capacity, and reduce the need for hospitalization.

Afterload reduction, angiotensin converting enzyme inhibitors

Afterload reduction with ACE inhibitors can increase cardiac output by as much as 30%. This happens without an increase in myocardial oxygen demand. It is one of those rare times that you get something (increased cardiac output) for nothing (no increase in cardiac oxygen utilization). It comes as no surprise that afterload reduction therapy prolongs survival, relieves symptoms, and improves exercise tolerance.

End-stage patients often are hypotensive. How can vasodilators—antihypertensive agents—be used safely? The answer is in the hydraulics equation (Ohm's law):

Blood pressure = Cardiac output × Vascular resistance

If ACE inhibition lowers resistance 30% and cardiac output increases 30%, there is no drop in pressure. However, if cardiac output is able to rise by only 20%, then pressure falls. The key to ACE inhibition in heart failure is to start at a low dose, and raise it gradually to either a target dose (i.e., lisinopril 30–40 mg/day), or until the patient develops postural hypotension. High dose therapy controls symptoms more effectively than low dose.

A number of patients have renal insufficiency. ACE inhibition is safe as long as there is no renal artery stenosis. Check serum creatinine a couple days after starting the drug; if creatinine goes up by no more than 0.3 mg/dL there should be no problem with ACE inhibition. A rise in creatinine suggests renal artery stenosis.

Low serum sodium accompanies high plasma renin activity in CHF (whether one causes the other is uncertain). It is also a marker of poor prognosis. ACE inhibition is safe, but those with high renin are especially sensitive to it. Thus, when sodium is low, start with a low dose (i.e., 2.5 mg lisinopril/day), and titrate the dose slowly.

Those who are volume depleted after aggressive diuresis may develop hypotension with ACE inhibitors. If that seems a possibility (especially when an initial trial of ACE inhibition caused hypotension), give the patient a "diuretic holiday" for a day or two before starting—or retrying—ACE inhibitors.

Cough complicates ACE inhibition in 10% to 15% of patients. It will not resolve with time, and the drug should be stopped. As therapy for CHF, angiotension II blockers have similar efficacy and do not cause cough.

Angiotensin receptor blockers—Cough is a common complication of ACE inhibitor therapy, and is related to potentiation of bradykinin. When that occurs, the ACE inhibitor should be stopped.

Comparative trials have found that angiotensin receptor blockers (ARB) (ibesartan, candesartan, losartan, valsartan, etc.)

are as effective. In fact, a recent trial found that adding valsartan to ACE inhibitor therapy reduced symptoms and a need for hospitalization (6). Even with ACE inhibition, angiotensin II levels remain high in patients with CHF, probably because angiotensin II can be generated through other pathways (such as the chymase system). You may consider addition of an ARB to ACE inhibition when blood pressure is not low.

A caveat: Val-HeFT found that triple therapy with ACE inhibition, ARB, and a beta blocker was not well tolerated, and suggested using just 2 of the 3 agents.

Why not just use the ARB? Recent evidence suggests much of the beneficial effect of ACEI therapy comes from the potentiation of bradykinin and increased production of nitric oxide. Angiotensin receptor blockers do not affect this system.

Afterload reduction with other vasodilators—Hydralazine works but it is tough to use. A short half-life requires giving it four times a day. High doses are needed to achieve a demonstrable hemodynamic effect. The Veterans Administration trials that showed efficacy (V-HeFT I and II) treated patients with an average dose of 300 mg hydralazine per day and found little benefit in those who could not tolerate at least 200 mg (7). Side effects are common at the high dose. Furthermore, these studies combined high dose hydralazine with isosorbide 160 mg/day, and the beneficial effect may require this combination. On the wards it is common to see patients on hydralazine 50 mg twice a day; at that dose do not assume that you are reducing afterload (or doing much good) (8).

Increasing contractility—Most patient with advanced symptoms benefit from digoxin therapy. One trial attempted to discontinue digoxin in patients who were also on ACE inhibitors, and found a worsening of symptoms (9). While digoxin does not favorably affect survival, it does reduce symptoms and a need for hospital admission (10). Because of its narrow therapeutic window and renal excretion, it can be tricky to use for those with end-stage disease. Toxicity may develop with an abrupt change in renal function (e.g., with decreased cardiac output or excessive diuresis). You must be sensitive to the noncardiac manifestations of toxicity (visual changes, nausea, anorexia, etc.), and not hesitate to check a digoxin level with any change in condition. Efficacy is slight at digoxin levels below 0.8 ng/mL, and the frequency of adverse effects increases when the level is above 2.0 ng/mL.

Dobutamine relieves symptoms for those with end-stage congestion. Given intravenously at 5–8 mcg/kg/min it stimulates both beta-1 and beta-2 receptors, increases cardiac output, reduces pulmonary capillary wedge pressure, and lowers both systemic and pulmonary resistance, without raising heart rate. The selective action of this and other catecholamines are lost at higher doses. An alternative is intravenous **milrinone** (0.3–0.8 mcg/kg/min).

Home therapy is possible with either of these agents with supervision by a visiting nurse; most hospice programs have experience with it. One approach is to determine an effective dose in hospital with hemodynamic monitoring. If pulmonary artery pressure monitoring is not feasible, an effective dose may be identified by observing heart rate, blood pressure, urine output, and symptoms. The minimally effective dose is used at home, with 6-hour infusions one to four times a week. Beneficial effects have been shown to persist for some time after the 6-hour infusion. Many patients experience a steady improvement in symptoms, and can reduce the frequency of treatments. Treatment just once or twice a week may help.

There is concern that catecholamine therapy may provoke ventricular arrhythmias in the face of depressed LV function. The risk of this appears relatively low as long as the dose of dobutamine is kept low enough to avoid an increase in heart rate. A patient who experiences a marked increase in heart rate with even low dose dobutamine may do better with milrinone.

Beta adrenergic blockade—Traditional therapies for CHF have involved manipulation of preload, afterload, and contractility. Over the last decade we have learned that the neurohormones secreted to compensate for low cardiac output have adverse myocardial effects. Patients with CHF have elevated catecholamine and aldosterone levels, and both—at persistently high levels—have myocardial toxicity.

Beta blocker therapy reduces mortality and, over the long run, leads to better exercise tolerance and reduced congestion. The earlier trials of beta blockade included patients with class II–III CHF. More recently, a trial of carvedilol therapy for class IV CHF showed a reduction in mortality and frequency of hospitalization for congestion (11). In this study, patients were excluded with systolic blood pressure below 85 mm Hg or heart rate lower than 68 beats per minute. The initial dose of carvedilol is 3.125 mg twice a day, increased at 2-week intervals to a target of 25 mg twice a day. Metoprolol is a good alternative (target dose, 200 mg/day).

Spironolactone—In addition to reducing mortality, the Randomized Aldactone Evaluation Study (RALES) trial found improved symptoms with spironolactone 25 mg per day (12). Patients with class IV CHF improved, as did others with less severe symptoms. At this low dose, hyperkalemia was uncommon, especially when the creatinine was below 2 mg/dL.

The benefits of therapy could not be related to either hemodynamic changes or diuresis. Instead, reduced mortality and a 35% reduction in hospitalization for worsening heart failure were attributed to the ability of spironolactone to reduce myocardial and vascular fibrosis.

Diuretics—Congestion, either systemic or pulmonary, is the most problematic symptom with end-stage CHF (Table 3-2). Diuretic resistance is common (13). Most patients with end-stage disease are on loop diuretics, usually furosemide (Lasix). It has been around a long time, we all have experience with it, and it is inexpensive.

Lasix resistance is common. Bioavailability varies. On average, about 50% of an oral dose is absorbed, but the range is 10% to 90%, making it difficult to know how much a particular patient is getting. We solve this by gradually increasing the dose until there is diuresis. The rate of absorption is slowed in heart failure, even more when there is splanchnic edema, so the effective dose may vary with the patient's condition.

TABLE 3-2	*Diuretics*			

| | | | Elimination Half-life (Hr) | |
Drug (Equivalent dose)	**Oral Absorption (%)**	**Normal**	**Renal Insufficiency**	**CHF**
Furosemide (Lasix, 40 mg)	10–100%	1.5–2	2.8	2.7
Bumetanide (Bumex, 1 mg)	80–100%	1	1.6	1.3
Torsemide (Demadex, 20 mg)	80–100%	3–4*	4–5	6
Hydrochlorothiazide	65–75%	2.5	Increased	Uncertain

* The longer half-life is an advantage, facilitating diuresis. When multiple dosing is needed, the doses should be separated by 6 hours (more than with Lasix or Bumex).

The problem of variable absorption is compounded by reduced renal responsiveness to all loop diuretics in patients with CHF, by as much as 70% when compared with normals. Renal insufficiency further impairs delivery of Lasix to the site of action (there is reduced secretion of drug into urine in the proximal tubule, so delivery to the distal tubule is reduced). The net effect is "diuretic resistance."

The maximal effect with Lasix is achieved with a daily intravenous dose of 160–200 mg. At higher doses there is little increase in natriuresis, and the risk of tinnitus increases. A hospitalized patient with severe pulmonary congestion may need this high intravenous dose several times a day. The maximal oral dose is about twice the intravenous dose when renal function is normal, but higher still with renal insufficiency.

When a patient is requiring high doses of oral Lasix, you may assume that there is poor absorption of the drug. That is the time to switch to one of the newer loop diuretics, bumetanide (Bumex) or torsemide (Demadex, Table 3-2). They work like furosemide: they are secreted into the urine in the proximal tubule and act on the distal tubule. The big difference is that bioavailability with oral dosing is much better, with 80% to 100% absorbed even in the presence of splanchnic congestion or renal insufficiency. Both are metabolized and excreted by the liver, and the elimination half-life is not affected by renal insufficiency. However, renal insufficiency does reduce the secretion of drug into the proximal tubule, so higher doses are needed.

If you are treating the patient with intravenous medicine there is little advantage of Bumex or Demadex over Lasix. However, with oral therapy, better absorption makes them almost as effective as intravenous Lasix. When comparing the new drugs, the major difference is elimination half-life, which is longer for Demadex (Table 3-2). This may be advantageous, as there may be rebound sodium retention between diuretic doses. It is for this reason that continuous infusion Lasix has been suggested for severe congestion that resists diuresis (a loading dose of 40 mg, then 10–40 mg/hr, with the higher dose for those with creatinine clearance less than 25 mL/hr). The costs of Demadex and Bumex are similar; equivalent doses are reviewed in Table 3-2.

Another issue is whether to give loop diuretics once or twice a day, especially as half-life is brief. Early in the course of CHF, when congestion is effectively controlled with once daily dosing, there is no reason to give the drug more frequently. Active diuresis restricts the patient's activities. As congestion worsens, twice-daily dosing is usually needed. With furosemide or Bumex, morning and noon dosing frees the evening for other activities. Because of its longer half-life, oral doses of Demadex should be separated by 6 hours.

Using multiple diuretics—There is synergy between the thiazide and loop diuretics, and adding an oral thiazide is the next step for the patient not responding to maximal doses of a loop diuretic (Table 3-2) (13). Thiazides work more distally in the nephron, blocking the absorption of sodium that escaped the loop of Henle (and the action of the loop diuretic).

Metolazone (Zaroxolyn) has been marketed for this purpose in the United States. Hydrochlorothiazide (HCTZ) is more rapidly absorbed, has a shorter half-life (hours rather than 2 days), and is cheaper. For these reasons, HCTZ may be the preferable drug (13). With severe CHF the doses of HCTZ is 100–200 mg/day given in two doses. The dose should be increased with renal insufficiency.

An occasional patient resistant to loop and thiazide diuretics will respond to a potassium-sparing diuretic, such as spironolactone, that acts on the distal nephron. Although untested, there is a belief that it works well for peripheral edema. Clinical responsiveness can be predicted by measuring urine electrolytes. Low urinary sodium and high potassium suggest that potassium is being exchanged for sodium in the distal nephron (the aldosterone mechanism), and spironolactone should work. If urinary potassium is low, spironolactone probably will not be effective. The half-life of spironolactone is sufficient for once-daily dosing to be adequate (50–200 mg/day). It may take a couple of weeks before diuresis begins.

One additional benefit of spironolactone is potassium and magnesium retention. Spironolactone 50 mg/day raises serum magnesium 15%, possibly the best treatment for hypomagnesemia, as oral magnesium is poorly absorbed (14). Conversely, patients with renal insufficiency should be monitored for hyperkalemia.

Another drug to consider when the loop diuretic-thiazide combination fails is acetazolamide plus the loop diuretic. It is especially effective if there is metabolic acidosis. The dose is 500 mg intravenously.

Dopamine as a "diuretic"—At low dose, less than 3 mcg/kg/min, dopamine improves renal hemodynamics and is thought to promote diuresis. We still try it, but at least one study failed to document a benefit for patients with advanced CHF (15).

Morphine—When all else fails to control severe pulmonary congestion, morphine usually provides relief (Table 3-3). It is a venodilator, reducing blood return to the heart. Pulmonary capillary pressure and symptoms of congestion are quickly reduced. In addition, it blunts the anxiety that comes with severe dyspnea.

There is concern that morphine may depress respiration. In practice, with all but extreme doses, this is rare in patients with pulmonary edema (or with the dyspnea of advance lung disease, for that matter).

With training and experience, physicians do a good job managing patients with opioids. There are practical advantages in having hospice involvement when treating heart failure with morphine. The first is that "narcotics" may not appear to be "usual treatment" for CHF; hospice care avoids any suggestion of abuse. Another advantage is that hospice nurses regulate the morphine dose and monitor its use in the home.

TABLE 3-3	*Effects of Morphine in Congestive Heart Failure*

Effect	Comment
Reduced anxiety	
Reduced sensitivity to hypercapnia	There may be resetting of the receptor, providing one mechanism for relief of dyspnea. The patient tolerates a larger amount of respiratory fatigue—a higher PaCO2—without sensing it. There is less effect on the hypoxemia receptor, so it is unusual for patients to stop breathing
Airway receptor	Blocking airway irritant receptors may reduce bronchospasm, an action that has been demonstrated in obstructive lung disease.
Depression of respiration	A possibility with higher doses, but this is an infrequent effect of morphine therapy. It may be used without hesitation in advance CHF and obstructive lung disease. Appropriate monitoring is important, especially when initiating therapy.
Direct myocardial effects	None; there is little danger of myocardial depression and worsening of heart failure (which is why morphine is commonly used in cardiac surgery anesthesia). The major hemodynamic effect is venodilation, reducing preload and congestion.

A brief inpatient stay may help with selecting the right dose. A reasonable oral dose of morphine (Roxanol) is 2.5–5 mg, given at 1- to 4-hour intervals. Increase the dose by as much as 50% at 4- to 12-hour intervals to control symptoms(Chapter 2). Pulmonary congestion, which tends to be intermittent, responds well to as-needed dosing. Within reason, there is no maximum allowable dose. Raise the dose until congestion is effectively controlled or until there are intolerable side effects (e.g., excessive somnolence or a change in respiration).

Nebulized, inhaled morphine, 5–25 mg (the equivalent of 2.5–12.5 mg intravenously) is an alternative to oral or parenteral therapy. Morphine receptors are present in the airway, and there may be a direct pulmonary effect depending on the cause of dyspnea. The onset of action is more rapid than with an oral dose, with mental relaxation in 2 to 5 minutes. In addition, inhalation drug delivery is more convenient than parenteral therapy, depending on the abilities of the home caregiver.

Nonpharmacologic therapy

Salt and fluid restriction—Salt restriction helps, even though we have effective diuretics. Our heart failure clinic tends to use lower doses of diuretics for patients with advanced CHF, and I attribute this to more effective management of dietary sodium by its dietician. The goal is salt intake less than 2 g/day.

Fluid restriction also helps to control symptoms. When the patient needs more than 80 mg/day of furosemide, limit fluids to less than 1.5–2 L/day. Although still in clinical trials, *vasopressin antagonists* may reduce the need for aggressive fluid restriction. These new agents promote free water diuresis. Vasopressin antagonists also have vasodilating effects, and pilot studies have shown improved exercise tolerance (16).

Ultrafiltration—When other measures have failed, ultrafiltration relieves congestion. This approach affords greater hemodynamic stability than hemodialysis. Vascular volume is held constant and cardiac output remains stable, despite a decrease in total extracellular fluid volume. Electrolyte abnormalities can be corrected.

Ultrafiltration removes plasma free water, usually at a rate of 1.5–2 L/hr, and the usual treatment regimen is 2 hours daily, or every other day, until a target dry weight is reached. The demonstrated benefits are relief of congestion, reduction in diuretic dose, and fewer hospitalizations (17). Tradeoffs include a need for vascular access, adherence to a regular treatment schedule in the dialysis center, and possible further loss of renal function.

The frequency of ultrafiltration can usually be reduced, especially for those able to reduce free water intake. New agents that promote free water diuresis may reduce the need for ultrafiltration (i.e., vasopressin antagonists, see above). But our present experience is that intermittent ultrafiltration can help the end-stage patient avoid hospitalization.

Correction of anemia—Remember that oxygen delivery is proportional to both cardiac output and hemoglobin. An abrupt fall in hemoglobin may be expected to cause the patient with borderline CHF to decompensate.

Pilot studies have found that correcting *mild* anemia improves CHF status (18). A randomized Israeli study of patients with poor symptom control despite maximal medical management pushed hemoglobin from a baseline of 10.5 gm% to above 12.5 gm% with intravenous iron and subcutaneous erythropoietin. Over 8 months of follow-up the treatment group had improved functional class and LVEF, and a decrease in diuretic requirement.

With these results we may expect larger, multicenter trials to assess the role of mild anemia in the natural history of CHF. In the meantime, my threshold for treating mild anemia is lower.

Exercise and rest—Aerobic exercise is considered good for patients with heart disease, even those with CHF. But studies showing benefits and safety have been limited to patients with class II and III symptoms. We do not hesitate to recommend modest aerobic exercise for those with more advanced CHF, but caution patients not to push to the point of exhaustion or severe dyspnea. Most with severe congestion, particularly those with resistant peripheral edema, are unable to walk enough to achieve a training effect. Nevertheless, we believe that an ability to remain functional requires regular activity. Fortunately, available data indicate that low-level exercise is safe for those with advanced CHF.

Extra rest also helps. Studies of alcoholic cardiomyopathy in the 1960s showed improvement with chronic bed rest. Enforced abstinence accounted for much of the benefit. Nevertheless, an afternoon nap with feet elevated is still a good recommendation for patients with class III–IV CHF.

Extreme Symptoms in the Terminal Patient

Many with CHF have ventricular fibrillation and die suddenly. Others die from "heart failure," and may come to the emergency room with pulmonary edema that is refractory to intravenous diuretics.

It is unfortunate when the doctor tells the patient and family that intubation and mechanical ventilation is the only hope for relieving symptoms. Despite a previous decision to avoid ventilator therapy, a desperate patient and family may have a change of mind, especially when this seems the only chance for relief.

An effective alternative that should be considered is higher dose morphine, titrated to relieve dyspnea. There may be depression of respiration with a dose sufficient to relieve symptoms. In this case the moral imperative is to provide relief of suffering for the dying patient, even if high-dose morphine contributes to more rapid death. There is no culpability. This is not assisted suicide or euthanasia, but rather necessary therapy for extreme symptoms (19).

Coronary Artery Disease
Natural History, Prognosis, and Clinical Decisions

The number of cardiac deaths over the past decade has been relatively constant at 750,000 per year (in the United States), and CAD is responsible for 60% of them. This is a disease of both middle and old age. Almost half of myocardial infarction (MI) occurs in people younger than 65 years old; 40% of men and 30% of women who die of CAD are younger than 55 years old (20).

About one-third of them die suddenly. Others develop ischemic cardiomyopathy and/or a chronic angina syndrome. They are faced with a decision between revascularization and medical therapy.

Notice that I said "medical therapy" and not "palliation." A remarkable development of the last 2 decades has been the emergence of medical therapies that favorably affect survival as well as symptoms. Patients with *stable* angina do as well with medical therapy as with revascularization, and this holds true for those with multivessel CAD (21). Those with unstable coronary syndromes, either unstable angina or non-Q MI, fare better with a more aggressive approach including coronary angiography and revascularization. But even patients with unstable angina often respond to medical therapy.

Prognosis—The risk of dying with CAD is related to a number of clinical variables (Table 3-4). The most important is *LV function*. Patients with low LVEF, and particularly those with clinical congestive heart failure, have the highest mortality risk. Do not underestimate the importance of symptoms. LVEF is good as a rough guide, but may not be that predictive for the individual patient. It is common for a patient with LVEF less than 20% to have good exercise tolerance and few symptoms, while another with LVEF 30% has CHF. The experienced heart surgeon, when presented a high-risk patient with low LVEF, knows to ask whether there are symptoms of CHF. If there are none, the patient has a fair chance of surviving heart surgery. Those with ischemic cardiomyopathy who have symptomatic ischemia plus CHF have the worse prognosis with both medical and surgical therapy.

TABLE 3-4	*Prognosis in Patients with Coronary Artery Disease (CAD)*

Indicator of Poor Prognosis	Comment
Congestive heart failure	Clinical CHF may be a better predictor than LV ejection fraction, and there is not always a correlation between ejection fraction and symptoms (Table 3-1).
Poor LV function	Including low LV ejection fraction and high LV diastolic pressure.
Unstable angina or non-Q wave MI	Those with these "unstable coronary syndromes" are at high risk for myocardial infarction (MI) in the near future.
History of multiple MI	Myocardial injury is cumulative. The risk of death with second MI is much higher than it is with the first.
Multivessel CAD	Those with single vessel disease and completed MI are quite stable and rarely symptomatic.
Diabetes, advanced age, or female sex	With each, the prognosis is worse with acute MI and with coronary bypass surgery.
Comorbidities	Patients with multiple illnesses do poorly (including obesity, and advanced lung, kidney, liver, neurological, and other diseases).

The *clinical syndrome* also predicts outcome. Chronic stable angina tends to remain just that (chronic and stable). The short-term outlook is worse for unstable angina pectoris (USAP, defined as new onset or accelerating symptoms, angina at rest, or prolonged spells). A British study of patients with USAP who were on an 8-month waiting list for elective angiography found that 57% had either MI or prolonged pain requiring hospital admission (22). We also know that a majority of patients with MI have a prodrome of USAP, with symptoms often not recognized as angina.

Non-Q wave MI has similar pathophysiology and is often included with USAP in studies of "unstable coronary syndromes." These patients generally have a tightly stenosed artery with ragged plaque surface, and are prone to occlusion and "completion" of infarction. In fact, early studies of non-Q MI found that the 1-year prognosis is as bad as it is with larger, Q-wave MI. Though early survival was better with the non-Q wave MI, reinfarction allowed them to catch up over the next few months.

Coronary anatomy also determines prognosis. Multivessel CAD and left main coronary stenosis are much higher risk than more limited disease. Interestingly, a totally occluded artery is more stable than a stenosed vessel. Think about it. You can be sure what will happen with the occluded vessel that is supplied by collaterals. It will remain occluded and distal flow will be stable if the vessel supplying the collaterals is not diseased. However, a stenosed coronary artery is unpredictable, as there is a risk of occlusion and MI.

Vessel size and extent of plaque determine whether revascularization is possible. Surgeons speak of the quality of the "target." Big arteries with discrete lesions are easier to bypass or fix with angioplasty/stenting. Small vessels or those with diffuse disease may be impossible to fix. Patients who redevelop angina after bypass surgery may have open grafts to big vessels, with angina coming from diseased small arteries. In such cases repeat surgery will not work. Trying to "palliate" such vessels with angioplasty is rarely successful.

Clinical decisions—Note the earlier discussion of revascularization for patients with CHF.

Coronary disease, like other chronic illnesses, is eventually fatal. We commonly encounter a patient who has had one or multiple procedures who develops more angina. The key decision is whether to have another angiogram or a revascularization procedure. Revascularization may not be possible for one of many reasons: coronary anatomy that is not amenable, poor LV function, comorbidities, or advanced age. Older patients often decline intervention, saying "I've had enough."

At this stage in the patient's illness there is a shift to palliative medical therapy. Attempting revascularization when there is little chance for success can be disastrous. Fortunately, experienced surgeons and interventional cardiologists rarely agree to "giving it a try" when the risk is high. But they may not hesitate to take a worn out elderly person with favorable anatomy to the cath lab or operating room. When arms are being twisted, the patient must depend on the primary care doctor and family to protect her interests (Chapter 1).

What I Tell the Patient

The sample conversation in Box 3-2, and the related discussion apply to patients with CAD as well as those with CHF. In practice, most of those with end-stage CAD have ischemic cardiomyopathy, with symptoms of heart failure as well as angina.

We do not mislead the patient when asserting the benefits of medical therapy. A decision to avoid mechanical therapies is not the equivalent of saying "there is nothing we can do." It is more realistic to tell the patient, "In your case medical therapy is superior to surgery." Emphasize that this is not the same as giving up.

I point out that as medicine is adjusted symptoms usually improve. Even unstable angina may be expected to settle down with medical therapy. "Nature does not like sharp corners or instability," and USAP tends to improve with time as collateral flow matures or roughened endothelium heals.

I am being honest when I tell a patient that prognosis is not predictable. This illness is not like metastatic lung cancer. Heart attack and death are possible, and it is important to have the family's business in order. But as is the case with CHF, I indicate that we could still be seeing each other in clinic for many years hence.

Palliative Care for End-Stage Coronary Artery Disease

Drug therapy

Nitrates—Many of the drugs used to treat CAD prolong survival as well as control symptoms. Nitroglycerin is an exception, as it has not been found to affect prognosis or prevent MI. It is a mainstay of palliation, both in its short- and long-acting forms.

Sublingual nitroglycerin works promptly to relieve angina. Patients often have the misconception that it is a "pain pill," and are reluctant to use it often for fear of "getting hooked." Whenever I prescribe it, I review its action as a vasodilator and point out that it relieves angina by improving the heart's oxygen supply-demand situation. Since it interrupts ischemia it is best to use nitro early, and not to wait for the pain to be severe. In fact, ambulatory ST segment monitoring studies have shown that most patients have had ischemia (ST segment depression) for 3 to 5 minutes before angina begins.

Sublingual nitroglycerin works for about 20 minutes. Taking it just before an activity that usually causes angina is a good practice. A patient on long-acting nitrates can do this safely, as there is just a 20-minute bump in the blood level that will relieve or prevent symptoms.

All of the long-acting preparations work. Some patients prefer nitroglycerin patches to oral isosorbide mono or dinitrate. Tolerance is a problem with all of the long-acting nitrates, and there must be a 10-hour nitrate free interval daily. This is usually done overnight, although an occasional patient with nocturnal symptoms chooses a morning "patch-off" pattern. An obvious problem with interrupting nitrates each day is angina during the nitrate-free interval. Adding drug(s) from another class often works, and you may time other therapy for a maximum effect when nitro is absent.

Calcium channel blockers—In most texts, calcium blockers are at the end of the list when considering antianginal therapy, as they have not been found to prevent MI or death. I move them up on the list when considering palliation, because they are quite effective in controlling symptoms and are well tolerated by sick and/or elderly patients.

Nifedipine is a short-acting calcium blocker that is a pure vasodilator; it should not be used sublingually as there may be an abrupt drop in blood pressure and reflex tachycardia, and both may aggravate angina. Long-acting nifedipine and other dihydropyridines (amlodipine, felodipine, or isradipine) are safer. None of these drugs slow the heart rate, and are good choices when there is bradycardia.

Diltiazem slows the heart rate in addition to its vasodilating effects, and is a good choice when there is resting tachycardia. It is my usual choice for the patient with bronchospasm who cannot take beta blockers. Diltiazem has been shown to lower the risk of reinfarction in patients with non-Q MI (23). As a rule, drugs that slow the heart rate improve outcomes for CAD (including diltiazem, verapamil, and beta blockers).

The dihydropyridines have little adverse effect on LV function and can be used by patients with CHF. Diltiazem may be used with caution. Verapamil, however, should be avoided as it depresses contractility enough to precipitate pulmonary edema.

Beta blockers—By reducing cardiac work beta blockade prevents angina. It also provides symptomatic improvement and prolongs survival for those with LV dysfunction. It prevents sudden death for patients who have had MI. Both metoprolol and atenolol are cheap, and are my first choices for patients with CAD.

There are some patients who cannot use them. All of the beta blockers aggravate bronchospasm, although beta-1 selective agents (metoprolol and atenolol) may be tried at low dose when bronchospasm is not severe. Remember that beta blockade has a peripheral vasoconstricting effect, and may not be tolerated by those with severe claudication.

There is variable response to beta blockers, yet regulating the dose is simple. You may safely push the dose up until there is problematic bradycardia (do not hesitate to keep the heart rate in the 50s if there are no symptoms), hypotension, or wheezing.

Antiplatelet therapy and anticoagulation—Patients with angina at rest, by definition unstable angina, usually have plaque with roughened surfaces. This unstable plaque surface with exposed collagen activates platelets, and platelet thrombi contribute to ischemia. Antiplatelet therapy prevents heart attack and improves survival. It also helps with symptom control for those with angina at rest.

Aspirin has proven efficacy. Those with unstable coronary syndromes, including unstable angina, benefit from aspirin plus clopidogrel 75 mg/day (24). Use this more aggressive regimen when there is pain at rest or there has been an increase in the severity or frequency of angina.

It is common for patients with unstable angina to have symptoms improve after a week in hospital on heparin plus antiplatelet therapy. With time and anticoagulation the unstable plaque surface has a chance to heal ("reendothelialize"). Although it has not been tested in clinical trials, I have treated patients with accelerating or rest symptoms at home with a 1- or 2-week course of subcutaneous low molecular weight heparin. I would be reluctant to do this without hospice or home nurse supervision, realizing the increased bleeding risk with combination therapy.

There is uncertainty whether warfarin plus antiplatelet therapy provides additional benefit.

ACE inhibition and lipid lowering therapy—ACE inhibition is our latest addition to the treatment of CAD. There is angiotensin converting enzyme in the arterial wall, and blocking it has a stabilizing effect. The Heart Outcomes Prevention Evaluation (HOPE) trial found that ramipril 10 mg/day lowered the risk of MI, death, and stroke (21). The study was performed in minimally symptomatic but high risk patients. It also reported a beneficial effect on angina, an effect that may be greater in patients with more severe symptoms.

There is similar experience with aggressive LDL cholesterol lowering therapy. Reducing the amount of LDL, particularly oxidized LDL, stabilizes vessels, and angina improves. Like antiplatelet therapy and beta blockade, these treatments are palliative as well as life-prolonging.

Morphine—It is less common to use morphine for control of angina than it is for dyspnea with CHF, but it works. In addition to its analgesic effect, it is a venodilator, reducing blood return to the heart and therefore, cardiac work, a nitroglycerin-like action. While not required, I have generally recommended hospice when using morphine for angina (note the discussion of hospice for patients with CHF).

Treatment with opioids may not be needed long-term. As noted above, unstable angina often improves with time, perhaps as collateral flow develops. But once begun, morphine tends to be a chronic therapy.

Nonpharmacologic therapy

Address other medical conditions—The most commonly encountered is anemia. Remember that oxygen carrying capacity is proportional to both cardiac output and hematocrit. Abruptly lowering the hematocrit requires a big increase in cardiac work in compensation. We generally reserve transfusion for patients with hematocrit below 30%, a threshold that may be appropriately raised for those with poor control of angina. Other medical conditions such as severe bronchospasm or hyperthyroidism with persistent tachycardia may also provoke angina.

Home oxygen and smoking cessation—Although it has not been tested in clinical studies, an occasional patient has less angina when started on home oxygen. Some of this may be placebo effect, a well documented and important component of all therapies for angina (e.g., in most clinical trials there is substantial improvement in symptoms in the placebo group). Oxygen is easier to justify for those with low arterial oxygen saturation on room air.

We think of cigarette smoking as a risk factor for atherosclerosis, and wonder if it is worth the struggle for a person with end-stage CAD to quit. The argument for cessation is the immediate effect of smoking on arterial oxygen carrying capacity. Smoke contains carbon monoxide, and active smokers have elevated arterial carboxyhemoglobin levels. Serial treadmill studies have shown a fall in exercise time and anginal threshold after smoking two cigarettes. A person with advanced symptoms may note improvement a couple days after smoking cessation as carboxyhemoglobin levels fall (25).

Spinal cord stimulation—Two technologies have been used, stimulators implanted in the epidural space and transcutaneous stimulation (TENS) (26). Randomized but small studies have found improved exercise tolerance and decreasing frequency of anginal episodes. By reducing the number of hospital admissions, this approach may be cost effective.

The mechanism of relief appears to be a mix of pain reduction and interruption of ischemia. Spinal cord stimulation reduces the transmission of nociceptive impulse via the spinothalamic tract. There is also decreased sympathetic tone with reduced myocardial oxygen demand. Over time there may be improvement in myocardial microcirculatory blood flow. This technology is new, and further study is in progress.

Rest Therapy—One of my teachers, Dr. Julian Beckwith, taught me that a sensible treatment option for uncontrollable angina is reduced activity, a "bed-to-chair" lifestyle. This was a common approach before the 1960s, and at times it is still appropriate. There is no doubt about the efficacy of aerobic exercise for patients with heart disease, both CAD and CHF. But there comes a time when it does not work, and reduced activity offers palliation. Your elderly patient may prefer this alternative to open heart surgery.

References

1. Young JB. Assessment of heart failure. In: Colucci WS, ed: Heart failure: cardiac function and dysfunction. In: Braunwald E. Atlas of heart disease; vol. 4. Philadelphia: Current Medicine, 1995:7.1–7.20.

2. Cleland JG, McGowan J, Clark A, Freemantle N. The evidence for beta blockers in heart failure. BMJ 1999;318:824–825.

3. Otto CM. Clinical practice. Evaluation and management of chronic mitral regurgitation. N Engl J Med 2001;345:740–746.

4. Cardiac Arrhythmia Suppression Trial (CAST) Investigators. Preliminary report: effect of encainide and flecainide on mortality in a randomized trial of arrhythmia suppression after myocardial infarction. N Engl J Med 1989;321:406–412.

5. Cazeau S, Leclercq C, Lavergne T, et al. Effects of multisite biventricular pacing in patients with heart failure and intraventricular conduction delay. N Engl J Med 2001;344:873–880.

6. Cohn JN, Tognoni G. A randomized trial of the angiotensis-receptor blocker valsartan in chronic heart failure. N Engl J Med 2001;345:1667–1675.

7. Cohn JN, Archibald DG, Ziesche S, et al. Effect of vasodilator therapy on mortality in chronic congestive heart failure. Results of a Veterans Administration cooperative study. N Engl J Med 1986;314:1547–1552.

8. Cohn JN, Johnson G, Ziesche S, et al. A comparison of enalapril with hydralazine-isosorbide dinitrate in the treatment of chronic congestive heart failure. N Engl J Med 1991;325:303–310.

9. Packer M, Gheorghiade M, Young JB, et al. Withdrawal of digoxin from patients with chronic heart failure treated with angiotensin-converting-enzyme inhibitors. RADIANCE study. N Engl J Med 1993;329:1–9.

10. The Digitalis Investigators Group. The effect of digoxin on mortality and morbidity in patients with heart failure. N Engl J Med 1997;336:525–531.

11. Packer M, Coats AJ, Fowler MB, et al. Effect of carvedilol on survival in severe chronic heart failure. N Engl J Med 2001;344:1651–1658.

12. Pitt B, Zannad F, Remme WJ, et al. The effect of spironolactone on morbidity and mortality in patients with severe heart failure. Randomized Aldactone Evaluation Study Investigators. N Engl J Med 1999;341:709–717.

13. Brater DC. Diuretic therapy. N Engl J Med 1998;339:387–395.

14. Barr CS, Lang CC, Hanson J, et al. Effects of adding spironolactone to an angiotensin-converting inhibitor in chronic congestive heart failure secondary to coronary artery disease. Am J Cardiol 1995;76:1259–1265.

15. Vargo DL, Brater DC, Rudy DW, Swan SK. Dopamine does not enhance furosemide-induced natriuresis in patients with congestive heart failure. J Am Soc Nephrol 1996;7:1032–1039.

16. Krum H. New and emerging pharmacologic strategies in the management of chronic heart failure. Clin Cardiol 2000;23:724–730.

17. Fonarow GC, Stevenson LW, Walden JA, et al. Impact of a comprehensive heart failure management program on hospital readmission and functional status of patients with advanced heart failure. J Am Coll Cardiol 1997;30:725–732.

18. Silverberg DS, Wexler D, Sheps D, et al. The effect of correction of mild anemia in severe, resistant congestive heart failure using subcutaneous erythropoietin and intravenous iron: a randomized controlled study. J Am Coll Cardiol 2001;37:1775–1780.

19. Sachs GA, Ahronheim J, Rhymes JA, et al. Good care of dying patients: the alternative to physician-assisted suicide and euthanasia. J Am Geriatr Soc 1995;43:553–562.

20. American Heart Association. Heart and stroke facts: 2000 statistical supplement. Dallas: American Heart Association, 2000.

21. Yusuf S, Sleight P, Pogue J, et al. Effects of an angiotensin-converting-enzyme inhibitor, ramipril, on cardiovascular events in high-risk patients. The Heart Outcomes Prevention Evaluation Study Investigators. N Engl J Med 2000;342:145–153.

22. Chester M, Chen L, Kaski JC. Identification of patients at high risk for adverse coronary events while awaiting routine coronary angioplasty. Br Heart J 1995;73:216–222.

23. Gibson RS, Boden WE, Theroux P, et al. Diltiazem and reinfarction in patients with non-Q wave myocardial infarction. Results of a double-blind, randomized, multicenter trial. N Engl J Med 1986;315:423–429.

24. Yusuf S, Zhao F, Mehta SR, et al. Effects of clopidogrel in addition to aspirin in patients with acute coronary syndromes without ST-segment elevation. N Engl J Med 2001;345:494–502.

25. Allred EN, Bleecker ER, Chaitman BR, et al. Short-term effects of carbon monoxide on exercise performance of subjects with coronary artery disease. N Engl J Med 1989;321:1426–1432.

26. Latif OA, Nedeljkovic SS, Stevenson LW. Spinal cord stimulation for chronic intractable angina pectoris. Clin Cardiol 2001;24:533–541.

Chronic Lung Disease

John E. Heffner

Chronic Obstructive Pulmonary Disease

Chronic obstructive pulmonary disease (COPD) is the term applied to several respiratory conditions characterized by expiratory airflow limitation (1). Chronic bronchitis and emphysema are the most common causes of COPD. These disorders result from an abnormal inflammatory response to inhaled particles (most often smoking) and have in common damage to small and large airways, various degrees of destroyed lung parenchyma, and evidence of chronic airway inflammation. Chronic bronchitis begins in the small airways with inflammation that spreads to larger airways causing mucus hypersecretion, increased risk for bacterial bronchial infections, and airflow limitation. Emphysema is characterized by irreversible damage to alveolar tissue that reduces lung elasticity and causes expiratory airway collapse and airflow limitation. Most patients with COPD have a combination of both chronic bronchitis and emphysema to varying degrees.

Sixteen million Americans have symptomatic COPD, which accounts for 4% of all deaths in the United States making it the fourth leading cause of death (1). Unfortunately, COPD is the only leading cause of death in the United States that has an increasing—rather than decreasing—death rate. The World Health Organization reports that COPD produces 1 million years of life lost per annum worldwide.

Dyspnea represents the most common and troubling symptom associated with COPD and results from expiratory airflow limitation. In contrast to normal persons, a patient with COPD reaches the maximum attainable ventilatory flow rate with minimal exercise (Figure 4-1). Those with severe COPD reach this ventilatory limit at rest. Once the expiratory flow limit is reached, the patient compensates with increased respiratory rate and lung hyperinflation. This and the increased work of breathing cause disabling dyspnea. Cough and sputum production are the other major symptoms associated with COPD.

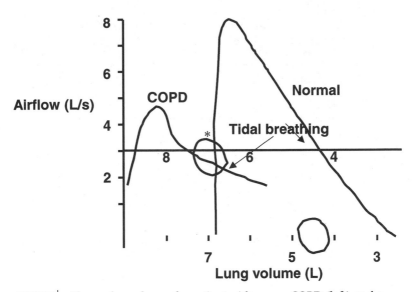

FIGURE
4-1 Flow volume loop of a patient with severe COPD (left) and a
normal nonsmoking person (right). The patient with COPD
has dyspnea because the flow volume loop generated during
breathing at rest approaches the maximal airflow that can be
generated by the patient (*). To achieve even this reduced
flow, the patient has to breathe at high lung volume, and the
work of breathing is increased.

Prognosis

The early course of COPD in most patients goes unrecognized.
There is slow progression of airflow limitation and a subtle loss of
exercise capacity. This is punctuated by acute exacerbations of
airway inflammation, causing increased cough and dyspnea.
Patients often misinterpret the symptoms associated with acute
exacerbations as being due to "chest colds." At this early stage,
smoking cessation is the only intervention that can prevent further
lung destruction. Eventually, symptoms progress and the diagnosis
of COPD is obvious.

Only 15% of smokers will develop symptomatic COPD (1).
Unfortunately, few predictors are available to identify smokers who
are at risk (Table 4-1). Moreover, it is difficult to predict the rate of
progression of COPD in those who become symptomatic. It is well
known, however, that patients with COPD experience a more rapid
loss of lung function as compared with healthy, age-matched
nonsmoking persons (Figure 4-2).

TABLE 4-1	*Factors Associated with the Development of COPD in Patients Who Smoke*

❭ Heavy smoking history

❭ Family history

❭ Increased airway responsiveness to inhaled methacholine

❭ Chronic mucus hypersecretion

❭ Low functional status

❭ Polymorphism in the tumor necrosis factor-alpha gene promoter region

❭ Elevated serum levels of fibrinogen

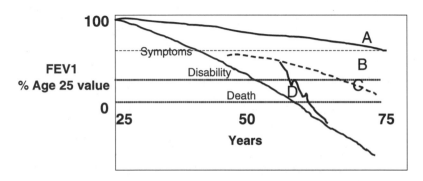

FIGURE 4-2 | Graphical display of the natural history of COPD as measured by FEV1 as a percentage of the baseline value at age 25. Nonsmoking persons with normal lung function (A) have a progressive decline of FEV1 but never become symptomatic from airflow limitation. Smoking patients with COPD (B) can develop COPD with a progressive decline in FEV1 that may produce symptoms, disability, and death. Persons who have lost lung function but quit smoking (C) have a decline in FEV1 that parallels a nonsmoking, age-matched person. Some patients with COPD (D) have a sudden decline in lung function with episodes of acute exacerbations.

Acute exacerbations of COPD also contribute to the morbidity and mortality of the disease. Patients with advanced disease who require hospitalization for an acute exacerbation have a 30% mortality risk during the next year (1). Those who are older than 65 years and who require intubation and mechanical ventilation have a 60% 1-year mortality. The presence of COPD also increases the likelihood of dying from other conditions, such as lung cancer.

Tough decisions for the patient with advanced COPD: life-supportive intervention versus palliative care—Most patients, as many as 90%, with advanced COPD who experience an acute exacerbation recover and survive to hospital discharge even if they require intubation and mechanical ventilation. There are some, however, who have respiratory failure as a terminal event. Mechanical ventilation for such patients offers little opportunity for survival, cannot reverse their chronic disabling respiratory symptoms, and only prolongs their suffering. In caring for these patients, caregivers face difficult ethical decisions about withholding or withdrawing ventilator support (2).

Unfortunately, physicians have limited ability to predict which patients admitted with respiratory failure will survive to hospital discharge if managed aggressively and which will not. Multiple clinical markers available at hospital admission have been evaluated as predictors of short-term survival (Table 4-2). Among these predictors, the baseline clinical features (severity of COPD and prehospitalization activity level) are the most important determinants of outcome. Multivariate models that employ these and other clinical variables, however, still incorrectly predict survival to hospital discharge in 25% of patients (3). Thus, dealing

TABLE 4-2	*Clinical Predictors that Predict Poor Short-term Survival with COPD*

Clinical features of this episode of acute respiratory failure
  Poor gas exchange
  Azotemia
  Hypotension
  Hypoalbuminemia
  Hyponatremia
  Acute physiology scores
    APACHE II
    SAPS

Clinical status before respiratory failure
  Poor exercise tolerance
  Advanced obstruction based on spirometric values
  Advanced age
  Excessive frailty or cachexia
  Significant comorbid conditions (i.e., heart or kidney disease)

with an unfamiliar patient in the emergency room, you cannot be certain about short-term prognosis.

Decision-making

Patient autonomy is the ethical principle that directs end-of-life decision-making (Chapter 1). Thus, the doctor must discuss limits of life-supporting care and the role for palliation with the patient who has advanced COPD. Experience indicates that most patients with advanced COPD wish to make their own end-of-life decisions either directly by talking with their physician or indirectly through surrogate decision-makers or written advance directives.

Despite the fact that assessment of prognosis lacks precision, it is fair to tell an elderly patient who has suffered one episode of respiratory failure, and who has a combination of the clinical features in Table 4-2, that end of life is near. In such cases, a person who has poor quality of life may elect to avoid future intubation and mechanical ventilation.

Many doctors voice concern that discussing these topics with a person who has advanced COPD will decrease the patient's hopes for the future and cause anxiety and depression. In actual fact, studies using anxiety and depression measurement tools demonstrate improved outlooks among patients who participate in end-of-life discussions. Discussion of the likely outcome of resuscitation also decreases the proportion of elderly patients with chronic health conditions who voice a preference for cardiopulmonary resuscitation by allowing them to form a realistic appreciation of the value of these interventions. Unfortunately, only a minority of physicians have discussed end-of-life care with their patients who have moderate to severe COPD. Consequently, less than 15% of patients with advanced COPD believe that their physicians understand their end-of-life wishes.

Most patients with COPD welcome physician-initiated discussions on end-of-life care. They also prefer that these discussions occur in an outpatient setting during periods of stable health when decision-making capacity remains unclouded by acute complications of their disease (Box 4-1). Respecting that a minority of patients prefer not to discuss these issues, caregivers should begin with an invitation, such as "Sometimes patients with COPD develop lung complications that require breathing machines and other aggressive care to save their lives. Would you want to discuss what we should do in various circumstances if you develop a problem like that?" Patients who initially decline to

BOX 4-1 | *A doctor discusses advance planning with a patient with COPD**

"As you can see, we are doing a lot of things to improve your symptoms from COPD. All of these treatments—and some we haven't yet started—are available to make you feel better and allow you to enjoy life. But none of them can reverse your lung condition. You should recall that COPD is a progressive disease that sometimes can produce sudden worsening of your breathing. We call this an 'acute exacerbation,' which may require hospitalization and sometimes necessitates placement of a breathing tube connected to a breathing machine to prevent your death.

"I am going to do everything I can to be sure you do not experience life-threatening worsening of your COPD. That is why you should call me if you start coughing more or having more trouble with breathing. But a life-threatening problem could still occur, so we should do what most patients desire, and that is to talk about what we should do if you ever experience lung failure.

"Some patients wish to have their doctors do everything that is reasonable to save their lives, including use of a breathing machine, if they develop lung failure from COPD. You would probably do well if you needed a breathing machine. If the ventilator is needed, I can give you medicines to make the experience comfortable and without pain.

"But there could come a time when a ventilator would not help you. For example, if you developed severe pneumonia, a breathing tube into your throat might not help you survive. In this event we might find that you got worse rather than better with the breathing machine. Most people do not want to 'get stuck' on the breathing machine, and prefer to have it stopped. When that is needed, we make the person comfortable with sedating medicines, remove the breathing machine, and death is peaceful. I emphasize that you are not facing a decision like that today, but bring this up so that we do what is right in the future.

"To do the right thing for you, I have to talk with you about the nature of these treatments, alternatives, and get a feel for what you and your family would want me to do in various situations. Let me give you this reading material on advance planning, and we'll talk more about it when we get together. If you have any questions, please call me. Also, our pulmonary rehabilitation program offers a wonderful workshop for patients with COPD who are making plans for their future health care. All if this is to help you put your mind at rest, put aside worries, and allow you to enjoy your life to the fullest."

---

* Note the discussion in Chapter 1 regarding such conversations with patients and families.

discuss end-of-life care often become ready later if they are provided pamphlets on advanced directives and decision-making.

It is generally recommended that the caregiver most closely involved with the patient's care should initiate these discussions, which has been called "captaincy." This caregiver often is the physician who sees a patient frequently in the office. Not infrequently, the patient develops a close relationship with another caregiver, such as a patient educator or therapist in pulmonary rehabilitation, or a home health nurse. Regardless of who initiates the discussion, all of the caregivers should be receptive, and ready to facilitate end-of-life decisions that are resolved by the patient and doctor.

Role of formal advance directives

Living wills and durable powers of attorney for health care provide opportunities for patients with COPD to document their end-of-life treatment preferences and to name a surrogate decision-maker in the event of incapacity (4). These documents, however, have had limited success in directing patient care during hospitalizations for acute complications. Moreover, many patients with COPD have an implicit wish for their physicians to "overrule" their advance directives if unique clinical circumstances exist. Recently, it has been emphasized that advance directives should serve as general statements regarding treatment preferences rather than explicit instructions for care that must be observed. This suggests that decision-making at the end of life is a shared process between patient, family, and caregivers. Decisions based on matching therapeutic interventions with the patient's previously expressed wishes, life values, and goals in adherence with doing what is best for the patient (beneficence) may at times override patient autonomy when patients lose decision-making capacity.

In this way, instruments of advance directive become less important as operational tools that list which life-sustaining interventions are requested by patients and more important as general statements of patients' comprehensive life goals. These goals, from patients' perspectives, center on preparing for death, achieving a sense of control over their lives, and strengthening personal relationships with friends and family. Physicians tend to see advance care planning as a process that selects treatment interventions; patients see end-of-life planning as a process that can fulfill their psychological, emotional, and spiritual needs.

Communicating with patients and families

The intent of the physician in initiating end-of-life discussions should center on fortifying family relationships and sharing decisions regarding life-sustaining care. Discussions should involve the family, with the patient's permission, and promote a dialogue within the family regarding the end-of-life events and decisions that patients with advanced COPD commonly face. Provision of educational materials and resources enrich these discussions. The emphasis of this discussion shifts away from selecting various life-sustaining interventions and toward developing an ongoing dialogue between patients, caregivers, and families regarding how personal life goals can be achieved and what realistic expectations exist for health care. Advance care planning is an ongoing process and should not focus exclusively on preparation of a written document. Patients or their families can make good decisions about end-of-life care when they receive comprehensive, comprehensible, and honest information in a compassionate manner.

It is important to reassure patients and families that treatment recommendations are not restricted to either "full support" or "palliative, comfort care." These modalities of care are not mutually exclusive and can coexist in the care of the patient with COPD experiencing an acute exacerbation. The patient should understand that the therapies used to prolong survival with COPD, including bronchodilators, steroids, antibiotics and supplemental oxygen, are also the mainstays of palliation, and will not be withdrawn.

Withholding ventilator support

When the burden of life-sustaining mechanical ventilation appears to outweigh its benefit, plans for withholding it are needed. The patient and family must understand that this is a shared decision so that doubts and a sense of guilt will not later emerge. This can be a positive experience if the discussion centers on *what will be done* to offer benefit to the patient rather than *what won't be done*. Thus, do not schedule a meeting with the patient and family to decide "what they want to do about intubation." Rather, meet to discuss the comprehensive care plan with its many options, including mechanical ventilation.

Occasionally, the decision to withhold life-sustaining interventions is less difficult because of the presence of overwhelming comorbid conditions, such as severe pneumonia and respiratory failure in a patient with advanced COPD. In such circumstances the doctor may exercise "unilateral decision-making," wherein intubation and mechanical ventilation are not presented to the patient or family as viable therapeutic alternatives because such treatments would have an extremely low likelihood of success ("futility"). In such circumstances, physicians must inform patients and families of the *medical* recommendation to withhold mechanical ventilation and request their support of the decision. Most patients and families will accept this recommendation although some will request that "everything be done." In such circumstances, additional discussions or a trial of ventilator support for patients with an immediate risk of death allow families and patients to accept the futility of aggressive, life-sustaining care.

In all circumstances, however, the decision to withhold life-sustaining treatment has profound meaning for patients and families, who often experience it as a family event that has no precedent. You should anticipate the fear and anxiety that emanates from this singular experience, provide reassurance that care will be provided in a humane and compassionate manner and that the patient will not be abandoned.

Once the decision has been made to withhold intubation and mechanical ventilation, a "do-not-resuscitate (DNR) order" is needed for hospitalized patients. This order may preclude all components of cardiopulmonary resuscitation for patients with terminal COPD or allow some (electrical cardioversion) but disallow others (chest compression, intubation) depending on the patient's wishes and the clinical circumstances. These "procedure-specific" DNR orders require careful communication with bedside caregivers to ensure that the patient's wishes are accurately implemented.

Some patients with COPD who forego intubation and mechanical ventilation may accept noninvasive positive pressure ventilation (NIPPV) by facemask (5). Noninvasive positive pressure ventilation provides the benefits of mechanical ventilation without the discomforts of an endotracheal tube. Patients with COPD and acute respiratory failure may be able to come on and off of NIPPV during the day. Also, patients dying with respiratory failure may receive symptom palliation with NIPPV. In discussing life-supportive interventions with patients with COPD it is important to explicitly describe the differences between noninvasive and invasive ventilatory support.

Withdrawing ventilator support

Bioethicists emphasize that there are no legal or ethical differences between the decision to *withhold* and the decision to *withdraw* life-sustaining care for patients who have reached the end of life. In fact, the moral weight may favor withdrawing life-sustaining care because of the added knowledge of prognosis derived from a therapeutic trial of life-sustaining care. It is important to recognize, therefore, that the ability to withdraw life support provides an opportunity to treat patients—and later withdraw the life-supporting treatment—when short-term prognosis is unclear.

Removal of a mechanical ventilator is the most common life-supportive intervention withdrawn from terminal patients with COPD. Patients may either undergo "terminal weaning" or "terminal extubation" (6). Terminal weaning involves the gradual decrease in the inspired concentration of oxygen and the amount of positive pressure. This gradual withdrawal of respiratory support prolongs the process of treatment withdrawal, but it allows monitoring for respiratory distress and sedation and analgesia as needed. Terminal extubation returns patients more quickly to their natural state without the encumbrances of endotracheal tubes and bedside ventilators, allowing a more natural death. Extubation, however, necessitates the anticipatory provision of sedatives and analgesics to prevent discomfort from the sudden termination of ventilatory support (6). Agitation or agonal respiration can be blunted with sedation, and this is particularly important if the family plans to be at the bedside.

With either approach, it is crucial to time withdrawal of life-sustaining care so that family wishes to be present can be honored. Families should be reminded to contact other important people, such as clergy or close friends, who might wish to be at the bedside of a dying patient. Attention to the availability of amenities (facial tissues, adequate seating) and aesthetics (the patient's grooming, collecting family pictures by the bedside) add to a sense of peace and well-being for the family. Consider the checklist in Box 4-2 when preparing to withdraw life support.

Relieving pain, discomfort, and suffering—terminal care

The therapies routinely used for the treatment of COPD, including bronchodilators, steroids, home oxygen, NIPPV, and pulmonary rehabilitation services, are also critical palliative treatments at the

> **BOX 4-2** | *Preparations for withdrawal of life-supportive care*

‣ Discuss with all members of the health care team to insure support for the decision

‣ Articulate the rationale for the decision within the medical record

‣ Anticipate the patient's needs for sedation and analgesia based on the medical circumstances and the patient's wishes (remaining alert or slipping into sleep)

‣ Identify one caregiver to communicate with family ("captaincy")

‣ Provide amenities by the bedside for family (e.g., facial tissues)

‣ Attend to aesthetics (e.g., grooming hair, shaving, bedside family pictures, removal of bedside charts, dressing in personal items)

‣ Turn off bedside monitors

‣ Remove unnecessary medical apparatus from the patient (e.g., cardiac monitoring cables, foley catheters, arterial lines)

‣ Lower bedrails

‣ Remove patient restraints

‣ Provide family members the opportunity to be by the bedside as support is withdrawn or immediately after

‣ Allow unlimited family visitation

‣ Allow private time for family to remain with the patient after death

end of life (6,7). When counseling the patient and family, emphasize that none of these measures that control symptoms and prolong life are being withdrawn.

Patients with COPD who choose to forego mechanical ventilation need additional, expert care to relieve their pain and suffering. Many of these patients remain alert as they approach the end of life. Ambulatory patients dying with COPD experience progressive dyspnea and difficulty with retained airway secretions. Multiple interventions are available to manage their associated discomfort (Table 4-3) (7).

You may be accustomed to thinking of hospice care as a service for patients with terminal cancer. But hospice is available and

TABLE 4-3	*Interventions to Relieve Respiratory Symptoms at the End of Life**	

Indication	Drug	Commonly Used Doses
Dyspnea	**Morphine**	
	Oral	5–10 mg q 3–4 hr
	Rectal	5–10 mg q 3–4 hr
	IV, SC	Titrate to relieve dyspnea
	Nebulized	5 mg in 2 mL normal saline q 3–4 hr with hand-held nebulizer
	Benzodiazepines	
	Lorazepam oral, sublingual, IV	1–2 mg q 1–4 hr
	Diazepam oral, IV	2.5–25 mg daily
	Midazolam SC	5–10 mg SQ then 10–30 mg continuous infusion (SC or IV)
	Chlorpromazine	
	IV	12.5 mg q 4–6 hr
	Per rectum	25 mg q 4–6 hr
Cough	**Opioids**	
	Codeine oral	30–60 mg q 4 hr
	Morphine IV	2.5–5 mg q 3–4 hr
	Inhaled anesthetics	
	Bupivacaine 0.25%	5 mg q 4–6 hr
Retained secretions	**Anticholinergic agents— recommended in unusual situations**	
	Scopolamine	
	SC	0.4–0.6 mg q 4–6 hr
	Transdermal patch	q 72 hr
	Hyoscyamine SC	0.25–0.5 mg q 4–6 hr
	Atropine SC	0.4 mg q 4–6 hr

IV = intravenous; SC = subcutaneous.
* These interventions are used when conventional therapy for airway disease no longer effectively controls symptoms.

particularly effective for patients with COPD who require specialized needs at the end of life (8–10). This care can be provided either at home with hospice service visits or through admission to a hospice inpatient service. Hospice nurses have expertise with therapies that affect pulmonary function as well as those that offer relief of pain and anxiety.

Morphine is as important in the management of end-stage symptoms with COPD as it is in managing the pain of terminal cancer (8). As a rule, patients with advanced lung disease tolerate morphine, and there is little depression of respiration at doses short of those producing general anesthesia. While physicians are competent to treat patients with opioids, having a hospice nurse visit the patient at home facilitates management.

Terminal care—Depending on the wishes and needs of the patient, sedation can be administered in a manner that meets the individual needs and desires of the patient. Some patients may wish to remain conscious to the end, others may choose to slip into "sleep" as their respiratory distress progresses.

In some circumstances, increasing the dose of oral sedatives and analgesics fails to relieve symptoms. Such patients require intravenous morphine for symptom control, and at doses producing "terminal sedation." Some bioethicists are concerned that the term, "terminal sedation," connotes an active intervention, blurring the boundary with active euthanasia (10). They prefer "palliative sedation" or "sedation for intractable distress of a dying patient." Regardless of the label applied, the fact is that the indication for treatment is control of extreme symptoms (which is the doctor's moral responsibility, see Chapter 1), not to shorten the patient's life. Intravenous therapy is given until symptoms resolve and the patient is comfortable. As long as drugs are administered with the intent of relieving symptoms rather than accelerating death, this form of palliation is legally and morally correct (10).

Patients on the ventilator who are having it withdrawn require special attention to prevent distressing symptoms. Although I discussed two approaches, I favor terminal extubation rather than weaning, as weaning prolongs the dying process (9). Anticipate dyspnea and treat the patient with morphine before removal of the endotracheal tube. Bolus or continuous infusion morphine and often a sedative are needed after extubation to relieve subjective and objective evidence of distress (Table 4-1). Assure the patient and family that symptoms will be aggressively treated, and that once treated there will be little discomfort even though the patient may look uncomfortable. Also point out that patients experience little discomfort from retained secretions in the upper way despite rattling respirations. Oral suctioning of these deep secretions creates more discomfort (and concern in the family) than the persistence of secretions.

In most cases, patients treated in this fashion die peacefully over a period of hours.

References

1. Petty TL. Definitions, causes, course, and prognosis of chronic obstructive pulmonary disease. Respir Care Clin North Am 1998;4:345–358.

2. Heffner JE. Chronic obstructive pulmonary disease—ethical considerations of care. Clin Pulm Med 1996;3:1–8.

3. Connors AF, Dawson NV, Thomas C, et al. Outcomes following acute exacerbation of severe chronic obstructive lung disease. The SUPPORT investigators. Am J Respir Crit Care Med 1996;154:959–967.

4. Heffner JE, Fahy B, Hilling L, et al. Attitudes regarding advance directives among patients in pulmonary rehabilitation. Am J Respir Crit Care Med 1996;154:1735–1740.

5. Meduri GU, Fox RC, Abou-Shala N, et al. Noninvasive mechanical ventilation via face mask in patients with acute respiratory failure who refused endotracheal intubation. Crit Care Med 1994;22:1584–1590.

6. Hansen-Flaschen J. Advanced lung disease: palliation and terminal care. Clin Chest Med 1997;18:645–655.

7. Rousseau P. Nonpain symptom management in terminal care. Clin Geriatric Med 1996;12:313–327.

8. Truog RD, Cist AF, Brackett SE, et al. Recommendations for end-of-life care in the intensive care unit: The Ethics Committee of the Society of Critical Care Medicine. Crit Care Med 2001;29:2332–2348.

9. Heffner JE, Byock I. Palliative and end-of-life pearls. Philadelphia: Hanley and Belfus Inc, 2002.

10. Heffner JE. End-of-life ethical issues. Respir Care Clin N Am 1998;4:541–559.

5 Renal Disease

David M. Poppel and Lewis M. Cohen

About 250,000 people with end-stage renal disease (ESRD) receive chronic dialysis treatment in the United States, and 90,000 start it each year (1). There is a remarkably high mortality rate, over 65,000 patients per year (2). Presently, 40% of dialysis patients are diabetic, and 30% are hypertensive. About one-third suffer from congestive heart failure, one-quarter from ischemic heart disease, 10% from cerebrovascular disease, and 15% from peripheral vascular disease. Only 9% of those starting dialysis have no significant comorbid conditions associated, while over 20% have at least two comorbid disorders (2). It is an increasingly elderly population; the largest cohort of patients starting dialysis in recent years is 70 to 75 years old (1).

Not surprisingly, the ESRD patient is often hospitalized, on average twice a year (1,2). Those older than 65 years spend 16 days per year in hospital for cardiovascular, cerebrovascular, and peripheral vascular disease, infectious complications and dialysis access problems. Regardless of age, in 1998, 25% of ESRD patients died during their first year on dialysis, and 23% during their second year. The first year death rate for those 65 to 74 years old was 32%, and for those greater than 75 years old, 47%. The usual cause of death was myocardial infarction, followed by infectious diseases (1).

Prognosis of ESRD

Patients and families deserve, and generally expect, a candid explanation of the implications of their disease. With ESRD, the available technology may serve to mask the potential burden of the illness, and clinicians should be careful not to instill false hope, especially among the elderly and those already deeply affected by the complications of diabetes and vascular disease. Such a hope may deflect attention from important decisions concerning advance directives and other matters relating to end-of-life care on the part of patients and their families.

The National Center for Health Statistics has published data predicting the average expected remaining lifetime for the US population in 1995 (3). These data can be compared with those predicting the expected lifetime for dialysis patients, based on age, gender and race (1,2). Consider these examples: A-25-year old African-American woman may expect to live another 50 years in the absence of ESRD, but the same woman on dialysis can only expect to survive another 13 years, and twice that if she has received a renal transplant. A healthy 50-year-old Caucasian woman can expect to live another 32 years, but only five years on dialysis and 11 years with a transplant. Finally, a 74-year-old Caucasian man without kidney disease will likely live another 11 years, but this number drops to less than three years on dialysis (there are no data on transplant in this latter age group) (1).

Several scales have been developed to assist clinicians in predicting outcomes for patients starting dialysis, and one of them is presented in Table 5-1 (4). Points are awarded for age and comorbidities affecting the patient at initiation of dialysis. Mortality is proportional to the cumulative score. Patients with a low comorbidity score (three or less points) have a mortality rate of only 3% per year, while those with a very high score (eight or more points) have a mortality rate of 49% per year (Table 5-1).

Communicating information about prognosis

General principles about communicating bad news have been reviewed in Chapter 1 and apply in patients with ESRD. We reiterate that the discussions often develop over a series of visits, and must be adapted to the patient's and doctor's personalities. While the nephrologist must be involved, the role of the primary care physician is critical because of longer experience with the patient. The influence of comorbidities makes it clear that dialysis has to be considered in the setting of the total medical history, a series of medical events experienced by the primary care doctor and the patient.

The discussion should include a review of all the patient's illnesses, and how the kidney disease developed. It helps to clearly define treatment alternatives, and to discuss pros and cons of each. Opening questions, like those reviewed in Chapter 1, are useful. Getting a feeling for how the illness fits into the larger framework of the patient's life is also important. The patient may have a specific goal, like living to see a child or grandchild graduate from college. Knowing this gives the doctor a better feeling for the decision process. Perhaps more important, taking the trouble to ask lets the patient know the doctor is concerned with more than just the illness.

TABLE 5-1	*A Comorbidity Scale that Predicts Survival for Patients on Dialysis Based on a Study of 268 Patients (4)*

Score*	Condition
1 Point:	Coronary artery disease
	Congestive heart failure
	Peripheral vascular disease
	Cerebrovascular disease
	Dementia
	Chronic pulmonary disease
	Connective tissue disease
	Peptic ulcer disease
	Mild liver disease
	Diabetes
2 Points:	Hemiplegia
	Moderate or severe renal disease (virtually all requiring dialysis)
	Diabetes with end organ damage (including renal disease)**
	Any tumor, leukemia, lymphoma
3 Points:	Moderate or severe liver disease (cirrhosis)
6 Points:	Metastatic solid tumor
	AIDS
Annual mortality:	≤3 points = 3%
	4–5 points = 13%
	6–7 points = 27%
	>7 points = 49%

* For each decade >40 years of age, 1 point is added.
** Thus, a diabetic patient with renal disease would have 4 points, and if 59 years old would have 6 points (with an estimated annual mortality of 27% on dialysis, assuming no other illnesses).

With this as backdrop, consider the sample conversation in Box 5-1. We realize that these sample dialogues are a bit artificial, and you would adapt this to the patient's circumstances. However, this gives an idea of points that should be covered, and the way that experienced nephrologists present them. Realize, also, that this would be a dialogue, not a monologue, and that the conversation would include questions that would lead it into other areas.

It is reasonable to mention that conditions may arise that could make continuing dialysis impractical. This is especially true for patients whose predicted survival on dialysis is short (on the order of a few years). Not only does such a discussion help put a patient's illness and prognosis in a reasonable perspective, but it

| BOX 5-1 | *A conversation about prognosis* |

"Mr. Harris, we have been discussing the possibility of dialysis treatment for your kidney disease, and it is important for you and your wife (family) to have some idea of just what dialysis can do for you.

"The main question is, 'How long can you live on dialysis?' The answer is not just related to the kidney disease, but to all of your medical conditions and your age. You are 68 years old, you have diabetes, and you have had congestive heart failure. The kidney disease comes from your diabetes and circulation problems. We have a lot of information about survival on dialysis which takes into account all of these conditions. For people your age and with your illnesses, the average survival on dialysis is 3 years. That of course is the average; with a little luck you could do better, but then of course, you could do worse.

"Another way of looking at survival on dialysis, is that your annual mortality rate is about 50% per year. By this I mean that of one-hundred patients like yourself on dialysis, almost half will die in the first year, half of the survivors of the first year will probably die during the second year, and so on.

"Of course, without dialysis, your renal failure would lead to death in the very near future, probably weeks or months, so dialysis certainly would prolong your life and could help you for some period of time. Given that fact, you may say to yourself that the choice is easy. But I can tell you that a number of people decide not to have dialysis. They figure that dialysis is obviously not magic since most die within 3 years, and that there is a fair amount of illness to bear during that time. Dying peacefully with kidney failure seems a better choice to them.

"Regardless of your choice of treatment, we will stick with you. If you choose dialysis, we will work hard to prevent or treat any new symptoms or complications. We also intend to help support your family as they deal with your illness, together with you. And we would hope that you could live reasonably well, remaining fairly active and free of unpleasant symptoms.

"What happens if you choose dialysis and it doesn't work out for you? Your condition could change so that you may no longer be living a life with the quality that you desire, and that hope for improvement is minimal. Just as you elected to start dialysis, you

Continued

> could also choose to stop it if you feel that continued treatment would serve no purpose beyond prolonging an inevitable downhill course.
>
> "The other treatment alternative, now, is no dialysis. In that case your kidney disease will be fatal, probably within a couple months. This is usually a peaceful death. Any symptoms you may experience are easy to control, and we would not anticipate much pain. Most people slip into a coma at the end. If this is your choice, be assured we will stick with you to be sure that you are as comfortable as possible."

allows the patient and family to understand that the clinician is aware of the potential for discontinuing therapy if it is not working. It also allows the patient to sense that he or she will have some degree of control over future events, and, finally, that the clinician is open to the discussions inherent in such decision-making. Candor in this regard also recognizes the fact that one in four deaths among dialysis patients have been preceded by discontinuation of therapy. Furthermore, despite end-stage renal failure, some patients may reasonably choose not to initiate dialysis support.

Deciding to start, withhold, or discontinue dialysis

Congress enacted Medicare support for dialysis in 1972, and since then the dialysis population has grown steadily. In the 1960s diabetes was a contraindication to offering dialysis, but it is now the leading indication for dialysis. A similar trend is seen with cardiovascular diseases that were reasons for exclusion 40 years ago.

The initial intention was to provide dialysis therapy for those who would gain the greatest benefit in terms of rehabilitation and long-term survival. Liberalization of acceptance criteria leaves a population of patients who increasingly have limited potential for rehabilitation and survival, and who may lead lives of relatively poor quality. For many of our patients, dialysis cannot interrupt the course of their non-renal illnesses, and "survival" on dialysis may only allow these illnesses to progress to the full expression of their natural history. In a sense, society has decided that any increment of survival is worth the cost, even for elderly and chronically ill people (for whom the results of chronic dialysis may be far from wonderful).

Over the past decade, the nephrology community has attempted to explore and enunciate guidelines concerning initiation and withdrawal of dialysis support. Representative bodies, such as the National Kidney Foundation and the Renal Physicians Association (RPA) and the American Society of Nephrology (ASN) have recently published practice guidelines (5–8).

Patients with ESRD have usually been ill for some time, and they understand the implications of ESRD and their prognosis without dialysis. Most elect a trial of dialysis, and they do so without pressure from their doctors. An occasional patient with slowly progressive chronic renal failure may balk at the timing of initiation of dialysis.

Although infrequent, an occasional patient will decline dialysis, deciding that an earlier peaceful death is preferable to a limited number of years with a considerable disease burden. This tends to occur with patients who have already had chronic and difficult illnesses, and especially with those who have a poor prognosis on dialysis. The clinician may re-present the data if the patient does not appear to understand the prognosis, and should be sure that the family has been involved. In the end, however, the autonomous patient has the right to refuse any therapy. The doctors should accept the decision with equanimity, and shift to a palliative model of care.

In cases of patients judged by routine criteria to be incompetent to make informed decisions, the clinician will need to rely on surrogate decision-makers. Again, the clinician is obliged to provide thorough information to assist the surrogate in making a well-informed decision.

Relative contraindications to dialysis—There are a number of clinical conditions for which dialysis is often felt to be inappropriate therapy (8–12). Most authorities feel that dialysis should not be started on a patient who is permanently unconscious, unable to relate to others or their surroundings and/or unable to cooperate in the dialysis process. Limitations of mental function that fluctuate and are possibly treatable do not contraindicate consideration for dialysis support.

Declining cognitive processes (i.e., dementia unrelated to uremia) provide a challenge that is best met by a shared decision-making process. This should include the individuals who can best assess the course of decline experienced by the patient and perhaps provide insight into the expectations or advance directives previously expressed by the patient. It is rare for a patient with advanced or clearly progressive dementia to start chronic dialysis. See the RPA/ASN guidelines for more help in this area (8). These guidelines emphasize advance care planning and the education of clinicians in palliative medicine, not only for patients in terminal stages, but for those on chronic dialysis.

A therapeutic trial of dialysis—The RPA/ASN guidelines also recommend a "time-limited trial" of dialysis for the patient with a medical indication for dialysis, but (1) with an uncertain prognosis, or (2) when consensus cannot be reached among the decision-makers (8). They suggest that the time period of such trials be determined on a case-by-case basis. Perhaps several days to 2 weeks would be appropriate in cases of acute renal failure, especially with coexisting acute medical problems with poor prognoses.

One to three months may be necessary for a fair trial for a patient with ESRD plus neurologic, cardiovascular, or nutritional compromise. In such cases, the question is the course of the non-renal illness, and whether it can stabilize once uremia is controlled. If the severity of illness and quality of life are not improved with dialysis, the patient and family may recognize the failure of the "trial" and decide to withdraw from dialysis. It is important for them to know that effective palliative care is available.

Discontinuing dialysis—The same considerations apply to the patient on chronic dialysis who is doing poorly. The usual cause is other medical conditions, usually cardiovascular or neurologic (13). When debilitation is severe, even the thrice-weekly visits to the dialysis center may be an excessive burden. The patient may have developed a new illness that changes everything (i.e., stroke with an associated mental status change). At this time the patient or surrogate may realize that dialysis no longer improves the quality of life and makes a decision to withdraw.

This decision is a difficult one for the patient or surrogate (14,15). It usually is not made abruptly, but is a decision that develops over the course of time. The physician may suggest the possibility, based on everyone's observation that things are not going well. It may then help to say that "we should not make a decision about stopping dialysis now, but rather think about it and see how the illness develops over the next few days (or weeks)." If the patient continues to do poorly, it will become apparent to all parties that it is time to either discontinue dialysis or to set other limits on care. These decisions are easier when a good plan of palliative care is in place.

Renal Palliative Care (16–18)

Symptom control is a staple of renal care, as patients with chronic renal failure, patients on dialysis, and those who forego or discontinue dialysis support are all likely to experience a wide array of unpleasant symptoms. Some of these symptoms will be related directly to uremia or dialysis treatments while many result from the underlying disorders that have led to renal failure or to comorbid conditions.

The symptoms of uremia—whether they be encephalopathy, anorexia, fatigue, pruritus, volume overload, and others—can often be treated by adequate application of dialysis, as well as related medical therapy (i.e., erythropoietin for anemia, dietary restriction, phosphate binders and vitamin D repletion for renal osteodystrophy and hyperparathyroidism).

Nonetheless, even patients on long-term dialysis who have been well-dialyzed can experience a variety of symptoms. These include intermittent hypotension, sleep disturbances, pruritus, restless legs and cramps, thirst, fluctuation in overall mental and physical function, varying degrees of depression, anxiety, and existential doubt. Spiritual and emotional issues and sexual dysfunction are common, and may not be disclosed to the doctor. Given the high prevalence of diabetes, peripheral and autonomic neuropathy are common causing hypotension, paresthesias, or persistent anorexia and vomiting (due to gastroparesis). Pain from peripheral vascular disease is not uncommon.

Aggressive and thorough attention to control of these and other symptoms is an important part of care of the renal patient. Though advances in dialysis technology and greater attention to delivering high quality dialysis have eliminated or reduced many symptoms, what is left requires palliation. Palliation should be applied across the entire temporal course of the ESRD patient's care, not only when dialysis care is withheld or withdrawn. Short of treatment with effective renal transplantation, ESRD remains a life-limiting, in a sense, "terminal" illness, and patients must be afforded all the benefits of palliative care.

Ultimately, this may include appropriate referral to experts in the field of palliative medicine. However, nephrologists and other members of the renal care team should be adept in palliative medicine. These clinicians, after all, will have the greatest degree of contact with these patients and their families.

Many of the ESRD patient's problems come from associated illnesses, such as coronary disease, congestive heart failure, diabetes, and peripheral and cerebrovascular disease. When this is the case, the affect of ESRD and dialysis on the clearance of medicines must be considered. Problems with overmedication may be as common as inadequate treatment of symptoms.

Practical treatment strategies for many of the most common symptoms associated with ESRD and dialysis are described in Table 5-2.

Sexual dysfunction

Sexual dysfunction is not uncommon in ESRD patients, and typically has multiple causes, including hormonal deficiencies, neuropathy, anemia, chronic fatigue, and depression. Discussions with patients may not only elicit a concern for this problem, but, by allowing a patient to understand the high prevalence of sexual dysfunction among ESRD patients, may afford some psychologic relief. Additionally, it will allow appropriate evaluation and referral for potentially treatable causes with psychotherapy, behavioral therapy, and medical or surgical interventions. Correction of anemia with erythropoietin may be helpful. In men, sildenafil, clomiphene, or yohimbine have offered some chance for improved function, as have certain urologic procedures.

Slow nocturnal dialysis may help sexual dysfunction as well as other symptoms (including hypertension, hypotension, neuropathy, and sleep disturbances). This is likely to gain in popularity and availability as it becomes better understood and more widely practiced.

Pain

Principles of pain control are reviewed in Chapter 2. It is important to know which forms of medications will best control each type of pain (bone and soft tissue, visceral and neuropathic), and to be able to anticipate and treat potential side-effects of analgesic medications. In the case of ESRD patients, special consideration to pharmacokinetics is important given the potential for excessive accumulation of drugs due to limited renal or dialysis clearance.

We have found that Ritalin may counteract the sedation that can limit use of opioid doses needed to achieve adequate pain control. More serious alterations in mental status, such as extreme confusion, hallucinations, or agitation may indicate excess accumulation of toxic metabolites or progression of more severe underlying metabolic or primary neurologic disorders, which may need independent evaluation and treatment.

TABLE 5-2	*Treatment of the Common Symptoms of ESRD*

CRAMPS

(1) Quinine 260–325 mg PO prn may be effective if given prior to symptoms (not to exceed 3 doses per day)

(2) For dialysis related cramps, hypertonic (23.4%) saline at 5–20 ml over 3 to 5 minutes, or 50 mL of hypertonic glucose (50%) may eliminate cramps, but the saline prep may cause thirst after dialysis, leading to excessive fluid intake

(3) Sodium profiling, starting with a sodium of 150 and decreasing in linear or stepwise profile may be helpful

(4) Serax 5–10 mg PO 2 hours pre-dialysis

(5) Carnitine 1000–2000 mg IV during dialysis has been suggested as useful, but not generally accepted as successful treatment for cramps (it has been suggested for myopathy, cardiomyopathy, and refractory anemia, though with little proof of efficacy)

(6) Vitamin E 400 IU po qd

(7) Muscle stretching and application of heat to affected muscles

HYPOTENSION–INTRADIALYTIC OR PERSISTENT

(1) Alterations in dialysis bath, temperature, sodium, and ultra-filtration profile

(2) Midodrine 1–10 mg PO tid or pre- and, as necessary, mid-dialysis

(3) Zoloft 25–50 mg pre-dialysis

RESTLESS LEG SYNDROME

(1) Initial trial of benzodiazepines:
Clonazepam 0.5–2.0 mg hs prn
Temazepam 7.5–30 mg hs prn
Triazolam 0.125–0.5 mg hs prn

(2) If benzodiazepines fail, try dopaminergic agents:
Carbidopa-levodopa 25/100 mg hs (higher doses may be useful if tolerated)
Pergolide 0.10–1.0 mg hs
Bromocriptine 2.5–20 mg hs

(3) Gabapentin starting at 100 mg PO qid and titrated up to 100–300 mg tid (caution with sedation in ESRD)

(4) Clonidine 0.1–1.0 mg hs

(5) In resistant or severe cases try opioids:
Propoxyphene 130–520 mg daily in divided doses prn
Codeine 15–120 mg in divided doses prn
Oxycodone 5–20 mg in divided doses prn
Methadone 5–30 mg in divided doses prn

NEUROPATHY

(1) Amitriptyline 25–200 mg/day, use with caution in elderly patients

(2) Gabapentin starting at 100 mg qod, titrated to 100–300 mg tid

(3) Carbamazepine starting at 100 mg bid and gradually increased in increments of 100 mg bid to maximum 400–800 mg daily

TABLE 5-2	*Continued*

NAUSEA AND VOMITING

(1) Treat associated hypotension

(2) Ensure adequate dialysis (KT/V ≥1.6)

(3) Antiemetics:

Prochlorperazine 5–10 mg PO, IM, or IV tid prn or 25 mg PR tid

Tigan 250 mg PO qid prn or 200 mg PR, IM qid prn

Phenergan 25 mg PO, PR qid prn

Thorazine 10–25 mg PO tid prn, 25 mg PR tid prn, 25–50 mg IM tid prn

Trilafon 8–16 mg PO qd in divided doses (not to exceed 24 mg/d), 5 mg deep IM with repeat in 6 hrs)

(4) Intractable nausea due to diabetic gastroparesis:

Metoclopromide 5–20 mg PO tid and qhs

PRURITUS

(1) Adequate dialysis (KT/V ≥1.6)

(2) Compliance with dietary restrictions and use of phosphate binders to keep serum phosphorus <6.5 and calcium-phosphorus product <60. Control of excessive hyper-parathyroidism.

(3) Epogen therapy as needed to maintain HCT >34%

(4) Correct iron deficiency

(5) Treat dry skin with emollients such as Aveeno Moisturizer or Oil, Eucerin Cream, Lac-Hydrin, Lubriderm Sensitive, or Moisturel. If response is partial, try emollient with anti-pruritic (e.g., Aveeno Anti-itch or Zonalon).

(6) In cases of pruritus only during dialysis, try switching to beef heparin.

(7) 2- to 3-week trial of antihistamine:

Benadryl 25–50 mg PO q 8 to 12 hrs

Atarax 25–50 mg PO q 6 to 12 hrs

Periactin 2–4 mg PO q 8 to 12 hrs

Vistaril 25–50 mg q 6 to 12 hrs

Tavist 2 mg bid

Hismanal 10 mg qd

(8) If antihistamine trial fails, start 3-week trial of UV-B photo-therapy three times weekly

(9) If that fails, try Naltrexone HCl 25 mg PO q hs

(10) If Naltrexone interferes with opioids used for pain control or is not tolerated, try Capsaicin cream bid to tid

(11) If that fails, try Ketotifen 2 mg bid or Ondansetron 4 mg bid

(12) If that fails, try cholestyramine 5 g bid or activated charcoal 6 g daily in 4 to 6 divided doses for 8 weeks

(13) If the above measures fail, try combination of antihistamine and UV-B light or cholestyramine and UV-B light

(14) Trial of plasmapheresis 3 to 4 times may be considered in severe and resistant cases

TABLE 5-2	*Continued*

INSOMNIA

(1) Ambien 5–10 mg hs prn
    Restoril 7.5–30 mg hs prn
(2) Evaluate for sleep apnea if clinically indicated

LETHARGY

(1) Ensure adequate sleep and assess for sleep apnea
(2) Ensure adequate dialysis (KT/V ≥1.6)
(3) Keep HCT 34% to 36%
(4) Treat chronic hypotension
(5) Encourage activity during day as tolerated
(6) If possible, encourage routine exercise program
(7) Encourage use of leg ergometer or bicycle during dialysis
(8) In deconditioned patient, consider physical therapy
(9) Encourage/assure adequate nutritional intake
(10) Assess patient's medications for those that cause sedation and decrease dose or substitute another drug
(11) Ritalin 20 mg qd

ANOREXIA

(1) Ensure adequate dialysis (KT/V ≥1.6)
(2) Assess for depression and treat with counseling and/or medications
(3) Treat nausea with antiemetics before meals
(4) Assess for gastroparesis or diarrhea and constipation and treat
(5) Evaluate and treat pain
(6) Ensure there are no mechanical causes that interfere with eating, e.g., swallowing problems, poor dentition, or ill-fitting dentures
(7) Treat disorders of taste with trial of zinc 220 mg PO qd and assess for and treat sinusitis and other oro-nasal infections
(8) In presence of dry mouth, try pilocarpine 5–10 mg tid or saliva substitute q 1 to 2 hrs and assess for medications that cause dry mouth and substitute if possible
(9) Trial of appetite stimulants:
    Megace 40–400 mg PO qd
    Marinol 2.5–5 mg tid
    Prednisone 10–20 mg qd to bid

PO = oral, IV = intravenous, IM = intramuscular, PR = rectal.

Meperidine (Demerol) should never be used by ESRD patients, as neurologically toxic metabolites will accumulate. Apart from this, other opioids may be used, and Chapter 2 reviews them. Generally, opioids need not be supplemented after dialysis treatments, but dosing requirements may be about half of what is necessary in the patient with normal renal function. This consideration should in no way limit the effective dose or dosing intervals needed to achieve adequate pain control.

Pain that originates from bone or soft tissue injury or inflammation may respond to non-steroidal anti-inflammatory agents which are generally well tolerated in renal patients. This is especially true with ESRD, when concern for renal damage is largely moot. A risk of gastrointestinal side effects remains, however.

Neuropathic pain may respond better to tricyclic anti-depressants, such as doxepin (10–100 mg PO qhs), trazodone (25–150 mg PO qhs), amitriptyline (10–100 mg PO qhs), as well as anti-convulsants, such as carbamazepine (200 mg PO q 6 to 12 hrs), valproate (250 mg PO tid to qid), and gabapentin (100 mg PO qod to 300 mg PO tid). Visceral pain may respond to anticholinergic agents, such as scopolamine (1–2 patches q 3 days), hyoscyamine (0.125 mg PO or SL q 4 to 8 hrs), and oxybutynin (5–10 mg PO q 8 hrs). None of these require supplemental doses after dialysis treatments.

Terminal Care

You may reassure your patient and the family that uremia, itself, does not cause pain. A number of other symptoms are listed in Table 5-2, and they usually can be controlled. Hospice care is invaluable, both for the control of symptoms and for emotional and spiritual support.

Families, caregivers, and patients should be given sufficient information to help them anticipate the signs and symptoms and the clinical course of the dying process. Those with ESRD often experience final days of high quality, in physical comfort and in their own homes. At the end, the patient usually lapses into coma and has what most consider a good death.

The authors would like to acknowledge Sharon A. McCarthy, NP, MS and Michael J. Germain, MD for their assistance in preparing the algorithms for symptom control in ESRD patients which, in modified form, are included in this chapter.

References

1. United States Renal Data System 2001 Annual Data Report, excerpts. Am J Kidney Dis 2001;38:S1–S247.

2. United States Renal Data System 1999 Annual Data Report, excerpts. Am J Kidney Dis 1999;34:S1–S176.

3. Ventura SJ, Peters KD, Martin JA, et al. Births and deaths: United States, 1996. Mon Vital Stat Rep. 1997;46:Table 16.

4. Beddhu S, Bruns FJ, Saul M, et al. A simple comorbidity scale predicts clinical outcomes and costs in dialysis patients. Am J Med 2000;108:609–613.

5. Moss AH. To use dialysis appropriately: the emerging consensus on patient selection guidelines. Adv Renal Replacement Therapy 1995;2:175–183.

6. Moss AH. A new clinical practice guideline on initiation and withdrawal of dialysis that makes explicit the role of palliative medicine. J Palliative Med 2000;3:253–260.

7. Moss AH. Shared decision-making in dialysis: the new RPA/ASN guideline on appropriate initiation and withdrawal of treatment. Am J Kidney Dis 2001;37:1081–1091.

8. Renal Physicians Association and American Society of Nephrology. Shared decision-making in the appropriate initiation of and withdrawal from dialysis: clinical practice guideline. No. 2. Washington, DC, February 2000.

9. Hirsch DJ, West ML, Cohen AD, et al. Experience with not offering dialysis to patients with a poor prognosis. Am J Kidney Dis 1994;23: 463–466.

10. Lowance DC. Factors and guidelines to be considered in offering treatment to patients with end-stage renal disease: a personal opinion. Am J Kidney Dis 1993;21:679–683.

11. Sekkarie MA, Moss AH. Withholding and withdrawing dialysis: the role of physician specialty and education and patient functional status. Am J Kidney Dis 1998;31:464–472.

12. Tobe SW, Senn JS. Foregoing renal dialysis: a case study and review of ethical issues. Am J Kidney Dis 1996;28:147–153.

13. Leggat JE, Bloembergen WE, Levine G, et al. An analysis of risk factors for withdrawal from dialysis before death. J Am Soc Nephrol 1997;7:1755–1763.

14. Wright J. On discontinuing dialysis. J Med Ethics 1993;19:77–81.

15. Lowance DC. Withdrawal from dialysis: an ethical perspective. Kidney Int 1988;34:124–135.

16. Cohen LM, Germain M, Poppel DM, et al. Dialysis discontinuation and palliative care. Am J Kidney Dis 2000;36:140–144.

17. Cohen LM, Germain MJ, Poppel DM, et al. Dying well after discontinuing the life-support treatment of dialysis. Arch Int Med 2000; 160:2513–2518.

18. DeValasco R, Dinwiddie LC. Management of the patient with ESRD after withdrawal from dialysis. ANNA J 1998;25:611–614.

6 Neurological Diseases

Jerome E. Kurent

Principles of palliative care are outlined in Chapter 1, and they apply to patients with advanced neurological diseases. For these patients, palliative care affirms life, and regards dying as a normal process. It neither hastens nor postpones death; it provides relief from pain and other distressing symptoms; it integrates the psychological and spiritual aspects of patient care; and it offers a support system to help the family cope during the patient's illness and in their own bereavement (1,2).

A devastating group of neurological diseases is characterized by chronic and severe weakness of striated, voluntary muscles in combination with total sparing of consciousness and cognition (3–8). The prototype disorder is amyotrophic lateral sclerosis (ALS). Other conditions include Duchenne's muscular dystrophy and related diseases affecting the motor unit, the locked-in syndrome and high cervical spinal cord injuries.

Patients with progressive dementia have cognitive impairment ultimately leading to a fatal outcome. Alzheimer's disease is the most common cause of dementia. Patients in persistent vegetative state (PVS) are characterized by an eyes-open permanent coma, and have no awareness of their surroundings.

Numerous issues affect decision-making and management of patients with these conditions. Bioethical dilemmas may arise during the course of managing patients with advanced or end-stage neurologic disease (3). These involve the ethical principles of patient autonomy, beneficence, non-maleficence, truth-telling, and social justice (Chapter 1). Some of these become clinical management issues and involve decisions about medical futility, withholding and withdrawing of life support, and responding to a patient's request for euthanasia or physician assisted suicide.

Diseases of Motor Function

Amyotrophic Lateral Sclerosis

Amyotrophic lateral sclerosis is a progressive and ultimately fatal neurodegenerative disease. The ALS rubric also includes patients with progressive bulbar palsy, progressive spinal muscular atrophy and primary lateral sclerosis. *Motor neuron disease* is the designation used in the United Kingdom for the ALS group of disorders. There are also infantile and juvenile forms of disorders affecting the motor neuron.

It is important to rule out potentially treatable illnesses that may mimic ALS in expressing the constellation of signs and symptoms of upper and lower motor neuron disease. These conditions include treatable spinal cord compressive lesions, such as meningioma, herniated nucleus pulposus, and spinal stenosis. Multifocal motor neuronopathy and other peripheral neuromuscular disorders must be excluded, in addition to other entities.

When early symptoms develop, competent neurology consultation is important. Because this illness is so devastating, confirmation of the diagnosis is often requested of a second neurologist.

Three-fourths of ALS patients die within 5 years from the onset of symptoms, with a median survival of approximately 4 years (9–11). The etiology of ALS is unknown, and most cases occur on a sporadic basis. Less than 10% of patients have familial ALS that is inherited as an autosomal dominant condition, and affects men and women equally. Defects of superoxide dismutase have been implicated in a small number of familial cases.

In sporadic ALS, men are more commonly affected. (The M:F ratio is 1.7:1.) The incidence of ALS increases until approximately 70 years. Median age of onset is 55 to 57 years.

There is presently no cure for ALS, and treatment is limited to symptomatic interventions. Most patients will die of respiratory failure due to weakness and atrophy of diaphragmatic and accessory muscles of respiration. Life prolonging interventions may be offered during the course of advancing disease, including percutaneous endoscopic gastrostomy (PEG) and ventilator support. Relatively few patients actually choose mechanical ventilation as a means of life prolongation. A PEG provides nutritional support when swallowing is severely impaired, and reduces the risk of choking and aspiration.

Prognosis

The rate of decline for an individual patient afflicted with ALS is relatively constant over time. The illness does not tend to wax or wane, and "remission" is virtually non-existent. Some patients experience rapid decline and die within 1 to 2 years, while others have extended survival in excess of 5 years. Those with rapidly progressive symptoms have the worst prognosis.

Patients usually present with asymmetric weakness and atrophy, often involving a distal upper extremity and then progressing in random distribution to affect all four extremities. The bulbar musculature is usually involved at some point of the illness, causing dysphagia, aspiration, or anarthria. Patients with ALS that only affects the bulbar musculature are said to have progressive *bulbar palsy*.

Amyotrophic lateral sclerosis is associated with clinical and electrophysiological evidence of widespread denervation, muscular weakness, and atrophy. Patients who present with bulbar weakness have a worse prognosis compared with others who develop bulbar involvement later in the illness.

Poor prognosis is often heralded by respiratory failure and, to a lesser extent, an inability to swallow. Hospice guidelines have been formulated for determining prognosis in ALS, and survival of less than 6 months is usually characterized by one or more of the following features (2):

1. Rapid clinical progression of ALS plus critically impaired ventilatory capacity
2. Rapid progression of ALS plus critical nutritional impairment, with a decision not to receive artificial feeding
3. Rapid progression of ALS and the presence of another life-threatening complication.

Communicating bad news to patients with ALS and other neurodegenerative disorders

Although the patient and primary care physician may have a long-standing and trusting relationship, the neurologist usually communicates the diagnosis of ALS to the patient. A second independent confirmatory neurological opinion is warranted if the diagnosis is less than certain.

It is helpful to ask the patient what he/she understands about the condition at the time of the meeting during which a diagnosis will be provided (note the discussion of principles of communication in Chapter 1). Most patients have little knowledge of ALS; it is often referred to as *Lou Gehrig's disease* in the lay community.

My preference is to avoid "dropping a bomb" on the patient, or "pulling the rug out from under" the patient and family caregivers. I have witnessed this blunt approach sometimes used during the early years of my career, and it was usually devastating to the patient. It would be sensible to guide your own empathic approach to breaking bad news based on how you might wish to receive bad news.

It is reasonable to leave room for hope. As noted, the progress of ALS may be slow, and at the time of initial diagnosis you cannot predict the rate of clinical progression. There is much active research, with ALS clinical trials conducted by reputable investigators. Most importantly, the patient must believe that you will be with him/her for the duration of the illness, especially when times are tough. Fear of abandonment is a valid concern of the patient.

The majority of ALS patients desire specific information regarding their condition, and especially their prognosis. A feeling of helplessness, which may be experienced by the patient and family as well as the physician, does not justify withholding information considered essential for the patient's future planning (3). This embodies the ethical principle of truth-telling, and which also has implications for informed consent.

At the same time, there is a delicate balance between providing immediate full disclosure, and the need for the clinician to communicate in a caring and empathic manner. It is often helpful to listen to the patient—how much does he/she wish to know today, in this particular setting? How much should be left for the next meeting?

One study described variability in the experiences of ALS patients who were first told of the illness (12). Some had a positive response: "At least I know what I have to contend with." Other patients were disappointed that they were informed too late in the course of their illness, or of getting the diagnosis without a relative or friend present. However, there are rare patients who might not wish to have a family member present.

Also considered undesirable were a lack of privacy (i.e., an open clinic or office area), getting the diagnosis in vague terms, or on the other hand, receiving excessive detail in a single encounter. These features of communication involve developing a delicate balance and sensitivity with the obligation to provide accurate vital information to the patient. This must be tailored to the patient's unique needs and personality appropriate for the circumstances. Consider the communication principles in Box 6-1.

BOX
6-1

General principles of communication when discussing ALS (or other neurodegenerative disorders) (12)

▶ Patients prefer the diagnosis to be communicated in a direct and empathic manner

▶ Patients and their family caregivers need opportunities to ask questions

▶ Patients usually prefer to avoid receiving overwhelming pessimistic messages all at once

▶ Patients and families need information on where to obtain additional assistance, such as patient associations and support groups

▶ Patients generally prefer to be informed of their diagnosis in the presence of a trusted family member or caregiver

Barriers to communication (13)

▶ Fears that the physician messenger will be blamed for the bad news

▶ Perceived lack of adequate physician time

▶ Lack of adequate physician training

▶ Fear of causing distress

▶ Fear of being asked difficult questions

▶ Fear of not being able to provide all the answers

▶ Invoking fears of one's own mortality

Advance care planning with ALS and advance directives

The living will and durable power of attorney for health care are the two most commonly utilized advance directives (Chapter 1). Guidelines for using advance directives in ALS have been developed and are reviewed with modifications in Box 6-2 (9,14).

ALS patients may inquire about remaining life span. Clinical deterioration is gradual with no abrupt periods of loss of function. Remissions are exceedingly rare, if they occur at all. At the onset of ALS it is impossible to predict how rapidly it will progress. A best estimate of prognosis may be provided later in the course of the

BOX 6-2

Advance directives for patients with ALS (and other progressive neurological diseases) (9,14)

▶ The physician is usually expected to initiate a discussion of advance directives. Such a discussion should be attempted with all patients.

▶ The discussion should involve honest and detailed communication between the health care professional, patient, and family surrogate decision-makers.

▶ The discussion should be initiated before there is severe advanced illness, or no later than when dyspnea occurs.

▶ The advance directives should be as detailed as possible about therapies and other interventions. It should include clear statements about life-sustaining and invasive treatments, such as PEG, tracheostomy, and ventilator support.

▶ The designated surrogate decision-maker and other family members should be closely involved in the process of delineating details of advance care planning.

▶ Cultural differences should be recognized and taken into consideration when discussing and formulating the advance directive.

▶ A health-care proxy should be appointed in accordance with statutes and regulations usually determined at the state level; the proxy should also sign the advance directive.

▶ Copies of the advance directive should be provided to the primary care physician, consultants and the hospital's emergency room and intensive care unit.

▶ All health professionals involved in the care of the patient, including nurses, social workers, clergy, counselors, and hospice staff should be informed about the advance directive.

▶ Once established, the advance directive can be periodically reviewed by the patient and proxy at approximately 6-month intervals.

▶ If the advance directive has a provision for a do-not-resuscitate (DNR) order, it is advisable to have a separate EMS/DNR sheet which should be placed at one or more conspicuous locations in the household, such as taped to the refrigerator or to the bedboard. This document would advise emergency personnel who might be summoned to the household that the patient has a DNR order, and that cardiopulmonary resuscitation is not to be performed.

▶ It is generally inadvisable for a patient to have both a living will and a durable power of attorney for health care. The two documents can be in conflict with each other. The durable power of attorney for health care is usually considered the preferred formal advance directive.

illness, based on the rate of clinical deterioration experienced until that time.

The need for patient and family support should be considered, and may vary with ethnic and cultural heritage (15–18). Antidepressant therapy for the patient may be helpful. Questions regarding suicidal thoughts may also be raised with the patient, and appropriate professional intervention provided when indicated.

Treatment of ALS

Therapy directed at the disease—Amyotrophic lateral sclerosis is incurable. However, riluzole has been offered as possibly life prolonging for patients with ALS (19). This medication has only modest benefits at best, and most patients will not detect any subjective or objective change in the rate of progression of their illness. Possible side effects include asthenia, headache, and nausea. It is expensive, and is not worth continuing if the patient feels that it is having no beneficial effect.

There is an extensive history of poorly supervised, irrational therapies for ALS including snake venom, chelation therapy, and others. It is important to advise ALS patients and their families about patient resources including the ALS Association of America, and appropriate internet websites.

Clinical trials—ALS patients frequently express an interest in participating in clinical trials. Ongoing ALS therapeutic trials may be determined by contacting the National Institute of Neurological Diseases and Stroke in Bethesda, Maryland. ALS patients should be discouraged from attempting unconventional therapies or those not approved by appropriate reviewing bodies. These may have the potential for harming the patient. Patients with ALS are very vulnerable to exploitation by unscrupulous pseudo-scientists and unwarranted claims for unproven therapies having no scientific validity. Patients should be forewarned to avoid these scams.

Palliative care

Shortness of breath and respiratory failure—Most patients eventually die of respiratory failure due to denervation and weakness of respiratory skeletal striated muscles. Patients with diaphragmatic weakness may complain of orthopnea. Other patients may experience increasing breathlessness when sitting up which may be related to severe abdominal muscle weakness and resultant downward displacement of the diaphragm. Portable oxygen may provide some relief. Eventually dyspnea at rest occurs with respiratory muscle weakness, indicating a need for respiratory support. This is usually associated with CO_2 retention. Acute respiratory symptoms may also occur due to aspiration, particularly in a patient with dysphagia.

Non-invasive ventilation can be effective in improving symptoms and $PaCO_2$. Non-invasive intermittent positive pressure ventilation (NIPPV) is the preferred technique, and has been shown to increase survival and to improve symptoms (20). NIPPV is a temporary solution, as respiratory muscle weakness progresses and non-invasive ventilation no longer works.

At that point, mechanical ventilation is required for continued life support, although most patients decline this intervention. However, there are ALS patients who have been supported with mechanical ventilation for several years in an environment of aggressive medical and nursing care. Most patients are unable to finance this, even if desired. Although some insurance plans cover extensive life-prolonging interventions, they often expire after a specified time. Families may then be subjected to lengthy and costly legal proceedings attempting to induce insurance companies to reimburse care. This often results in families being forced to use, and eventually exhaust, their personal resources.

Palliation of dyspnea may include the use of benzodiazepines and opioids. The potential risk of respiratory depression with these drugs must be considered, and close attention to dosages is required.

"Terminal weaning" may be necessary if the ALS patient decides he/she no longer desires ventilatory support (this is reviewed in Chapter 4). It is morally and ethically acceptable to withdraw mechanical life support if the patient expresses this wish (8,20). There are also legal precedents permitting this practice. The ventilator may be adjusted so that the patient is allowed to develop progressive hypercapnia with subsequent coma. Some patients may require the use of benzodiazepines or morphine to facilitate terminal weaning.

Dysphagia—Difficulty swallowing develops in almost all patients with ALS (14). The mechanism includes upper motor neuron pathology and pseudobulbar palsy. Lower motor neuron involvement of the cranial nerve motor nuclei innervating muscles of the tongue, pharynx, jaw, and face also compromise chewing and swallowing. Evaluation of dysphagia may entail use of fluoroscopic or endoscopic procedures.

Compensatory techniques may be employed to minimize the risk of dysphagia complications. These include supraglottic swallowing which facilitates the closing of the vocal cords during the swallowing process. The patient is instructed to hold his breath while swallowing, and then exhale at full force immediately afterwards. Postural changes can also be helpful. The patient may tilt the head forward, tuck the chin down, and then swallow (8).

The most effective intervention used to treat dysphagia is PEG. If there is an impending need for a PEG, it is advisable to perform the procedure earlier in the patient's illness to minimize complications related to progressive respiratory muscle weakness. The decision to utilize a PEG should be made only after careful discussion of risks and benefits of the procedure with the patient and family caregivers. It is advisable that the PEG be placed while the patient's forced vital capacity (FVC) is still greater than 50% of predicted in order to minimize risks of the procedure.

Sialorrhea and excessive mucus production—Excessive salivation with drooling occurs commonly, and is caused by facial weakness and compromised ability to swallow. Pharmacologic approaches to minimize salivation include use of amitriptyline at doses ranging from 10–150 mg daily. Special care should be used when using this first generation tricyclic medication in older patients as it may cause confusion or urinary retention (anti-cholinergic toxicity). Atropine and benztropine, as well as other anti-cholinergic medications have also been used successfully. Transdermal hyoscine patches are also used effectively (14).

Thick mucus secretions may be particularly problematic, especially nearing end-stage ALS. This may result from diminished fluid intake along with intercurrent respiratory tract infections. N-acetylcystine may be helpful for some patients. Physical therapy with vibration massages may be useful.

Muscle cramps—Cramps may cause significant discomfort for patients with ALS. They may be controlled with quinine sulfate 200 mg once or twice daily. Carbamazepine 200 mg two to three times daily may also be effective, but periodic monitoring of blood counts is indicated when using this medication. It is advisable to initiate therapy at 100 mg per day, and to increase by 100 mg increments on a daily basis to minimize possible side effects of dizziness. Dosages of 200–400 mg three times daily should be effective. Baclofen may also be helpful for treating cramps, at 10 mg three times daily.

Spasticity occurs in some patients. Baclofen may be initiated at 10 mg three times daily, and increased as needed. However, at higher doses the mechanical stabilizing influence of spasticity may be eliminated and may unmask weakness. Dosage of the medication should be reduced if this occurs.

Patients with ALS may experience subjective benefit from physical therapy, although this intervention has no effect on the natural history of this disorder. Pyridostigmine, an acetylcholinesterase inhibitor, has been used up to 40 mg three times daily for short-term transient increase in strength. This effect is usually of minimal benefit and should not be used on a regular basis, and only for specific situations, such as when taking an extensive trip. There is no rationale for long-term therapy with pyridostigmine in ALS patients (14).

Depression—Depression and suicidal thoughts are common in patients with ALS. However, suicidal intent is rare (14). Counseling and pharmacologic therapy of depression is strongly advised in symptomatic patients. Serotonin reuptake inhibitors or tricyclic antidepressants may be utilized effectively.

Sleep disturbance may occur, usually because of dyspnea, and oxygen desaturation. But it can also occur in conjunction with anxiety and depression.

Other common symptoms (3–5,21)—Constipation may occur on the basis of reduced fluid intake and immobility. Bowel regimens should be utilized including the use of stool softeners, stimulant laxatives, and osmotic agents, as needed (Chapter 2).

Pain may occur in ALS patients, even though there is no neuropathological evidence of sensory nerve involvement. Pain assessment is important, and pain should be appropriately treated. Minor analgesics such as acetaminophen and non-steroidal anti-inflammatory agents may be of value. Weak opioids may be indicated according to individual patient needs. Constipation is a common side effect of opioid use, and should be aggressively treated when it occurs. It is preferable to have patients on a bowel regimen if taking opioids on a regular basis.

Patients with advanced ALS may experience complete anarthria. Modern computer-assisted devices have greatly advanced the ability of the ALS patient to communicate. Eye blinking alone may be adequate to successfully use a computer which will create audible vocalization for the patient with ALS.

Related Conditions Characterized by Severe Weakness

Patients with end-stage Duchenne's muscular dystrophy and those with high cervical spinal cord lesions can benefit from palliative care interventions. Approximately one-third of patients with Duchenne's muscular dystrophy are mentally retarded, ranging in severity from mild to severe. This may potentially compromise their independent decision-making capacity. Family surrogate decision-makers may assume an important role in this regard.

Patients with acute traumatic high cervical spinal cord injuries may be severely depressed immediately following the devastating neurologic injury. These patients may request discontinuation of life support. That decision is the right of any autonomous individual. However, you might point out that the early, acute phase of an illness may be a bad time to make this decision. In many cases, those who delayed this decision or whose requests were not honored subsequently had an acceptable quality of life, and many of them were grateful that they survived beyond their acute injury. This poses a significant challenge for the physician caring for these severely incapacitated patients.

Palliative care of those with end-stage Duchenne's muscular dystrophy and high cervical cord injuries is similar to that of ALS.

Dementia

Alzheimer's Disease

Dementing illness is a major public health problem in the United States. Alzheimer's disease is responsible for up to two-thirds of cases of dementia (22). Most remaining patients with severe cognitive impairment are afflicted with multi-infarct dementia, or a combination of pathologies including vascular ischemic changes along with neuropathologic evidence of Alzheimer's disease. Less common causes of dementing illness include Lewy body disease, and neurodegenerative processes such as Huntington's disease, Parkinson's disease, and less commonly, multiple sclerosis and stroke.

Alzheimer's disease afflicts between 1.5 and 3 million patients in the United States, and is evident in an estimated 40% to 50% of all nursing home residents. The prevalence of Alzheimer's disease is expected to triple by the year 2050 unless effective prevention and treatment strategies are developed (3). Both the incidence and prevalence of Alzheimer's disease is expected to rise exponentially with the aging of our population. The fastest growing segment of the US population is represented by individuals 85 years and older. At least 20% of this aging cohort, referred to as the *very old*, is affected by Alzheimer's disease.

Critical bioethical issues challenge society and the physician caring for the Alzheimer's patient. The primary goal is to respect patient autonomy, and to provide the most humane and dignified care possible. There are also societal and related economic challenges which will affect medical and non-medical decision-making in the years to come.

These considerations include the realization that there are only finite resources available to provide health care to all members of our society; the relatively low value that society seems to place on elderly demented patients compared with other health care priorities; and our overall ambivalence toward demented elderly patients as a general reflection of professional and personal values (3).

Prognosis

The natural history of Alzheimer's disease is variable. Most patients will survive 8 to 10 years, with the majority requiring care in a long-term care facility during advanced stages of illness (23). Ten to twenty percent of patients may have rapid clinical decline and die within 2 to 4 years. The cause of death in patients with advanced Alzheimer's disease is usually a combination of medical comorbidities, or complications of chronic disability, such as urosepsis, pulmonary infection, or multi-organ failure. An inability to voluntarily eat plus the decision to avoid tube feeding may contribute to death (note the discussion of tube feeding in Chapter 11).

Communication and clinical decision-making for patients with Alzheimer's disease

The diagnosis of Alzheimer's disease should be communicated compassionately and in simple language (note the above discussion including Boxes 6-1 and 6-2, and Chapter 1) (3). It should involve the patient and family caregivers. Ample time should be provided for questions and discussion. It is important that all potential available therapeutic interventions and management strategies be reviewed, including participation in patient advocacy and family support groups.

The value of adult day care centers for family caregiver respite, and opportunities for clinical research may also be discussed. The patient and family should be assured that they will not be abandoned over the course of the Alzheimer patient's illness. This implies a serious commitment by the primary care physician.

Decision-making capacity—The issues of decision-making capacity and competency for the patient with cognitive impairment have been reviewed in detail (23,24). Patients with cognitive impairment may still retain decision-making capacity for specific focused issues (e.g., choosing a proxy; and even electing a do-not-resuscitate [DNR] order). The term *competency* is considered a legal term, and should not be confused with *capacity* when used in the medical decision-making context. Questions of decision-making capacity may sometimes be referred for psychiatric consultation for resolution, but this is usually not necessary. The hospital's Medical Ethics Committee may also help to resolve difficult issues.

Advance directives—The living will and durable power of attorney for health care help us honor the wishes of an Alzheimer's patient who subsequently loses decision-making capacity. Controversy has become evident under these circumstances, and have presented serious medical-ethical dilemmas.

A patient with Alzheimer's disease may have earlier declared a wish to withhold hydration and nutrition and other life prolonging treatments. This earlier directive may come into conflict with a subsequent expression of preferences favoring more aggressive treatment which is made after the development of advanced dementia.

Should the earlier directive be honored because the patient was competent? Does it possess more credibility when compared with wishes made subsequently after clinical evolution to advanced dementia?

Convincing arguments have been developed in favor of honoring the advance directive executed when the patient had full decision-making capacity. Other compelling arguments have been developed which indicate that the selfhood and identity of a demented person persists even when the patient becomes severely impaired from dementing illness. The role of surrogate decision-makers may facilitate decision-making in this very difficult circumstance. Such decisions may be facilitated by an ethics committee consultation.

Treatment of Alzheimer's disease

Acetyl cholinesterase inhibitors have been approved by the FDA for use in patients with Alzheimer's disease. Donepezil may be initiated at 5 mg daily, and increased to 10 mg daily if the lower dose is tolerated. This medication and related congeners have no effect on the rate of disease progression. In some instances they provide modest symptomatic improvement such as improved short-term memory. However, these improvements—when they occur—are rarely dramatic and lasting (22). The cost of these drugs may also limit their use. Gastrointestinal (GI) side effects such as diarrhea may occur at higher doses, prompting reduction in dose.

Palliative Care for Patients with Advanced Dementia

Some Alzheimer's special care units have implemented palliative care plans. In the US, Alzheimer's patients are often treated with antibiotics if they develop significant infections, such as pneumonia or urosepsis. However, studies have indicated that mortality rates comparing treated and untreated patients with antibiotics did not vary significantly in this patient population.

Although palliative care may benefit patients with advanced Alzheimer's disease, hospice is unfortunately rarely utilized (less than 1% of all hospice enrollees in the US). Efforts are underway to increase availability of hospice for patients with Alzheimer's disease. *A Physician's Guide* has been developed by the National Hospice and Palliative Care Organization to facilitate entry of patients with non-cancer diagnoses, including patients with Alzheimer's disease into hospice (2). Physicians may be reluctant to make appropriate referrals because of difficulty in determining prognosis. The hospice team can be helpful in evaluating patients for hospice eligibility, and consultation is encouraged for this purpose.

Alzheimer's special care units are useful for the patient with advanced disease, especially for those who have become combative, who wander or have other behavioral problems. These community-based facilities can also provide greatly needed respite care for family caregivers.

Functional assessment of the patient with Alzheimer's disease—
The Functional Assessment Staging (FAST) instrument is utilized to help determine hospice eligibility for patients with Alzheimer's

disease (2). A scoring mechanism ranging from 1–7 is used. Stage 1 indicates no difficulty in functioning, either subjectively or objectively, while Stage 2 indicates that the Alzheimer's patient forgets the location of objects and having difficulty with various simple tasks. Maximum disability is indicated by Stage 7, with subcategories progressing from A through F. Alzheimer's patients must be ranked at a scale of 7A or higher for hospice eligibility.

Comfort and supportive care—Comfort measures for the patient with Alzheimer's disease include the maintenance of good hygiene, such as bathing, grooming, skin care, bowel and bladder function, and re-positioning when indicated. Aggressive interventions including acute care hospital admissions and surgical procedures should be avoided unless there is clear benefit for the patient in promoting high quality of life. Prolonging the dying process should be avoided. The control of physical symptoms including pain has been reviewed in Chapter 2 (25).

Treatment for depression with selective serotonin reuptake inhibitors (SSRIs) may be indicated, especially for patients in the early stages of Alzheimer's disease. Neuroleptic medications, including low-dose haloperidol, as low as 0.25–0.5 mg one to three times daily, and can be increased depending on specific clinical needs. Risperidone, 0.25–0.5 mg one to two times daily, may be initiated as treatment for hallucinations and other symptoms of psychosis related to advancing Alzheimer's disease, but may have to be increased considerably. Anxiolytics, including low-dose, short-acting benzodiazepines, such as lorazepam, may be very helpful, and can be administered as 0.25–0.5 mg one to three times daily. Hypnotic agents, such as zolpidem 2.5 mg hs or 5 mg hs, or temazepam at 7.5 mg hs, can assist with sleep.

It is important to appreciate that neuroleptics, anxiolytics, and antidepressant medications may predispose to falls, with the significant potential for fracture and other serious injury. Medications must be closely monitored, and if necessary adjusted to meet the needs of individual patients. A good principle for treating geriatric patients and monitoring dosages is to *start low, and go slow*. Primary care clinicians not familiar with the frequent use of these potent medications are urged to obtain consultation from psychiatry or clinical pharmacy colleagues.

Tube feeding—The issue of nutritional support has received much attention. A survey of internal medicine physicians indicated that 84% believe that tube feeding of patients with advanced dementia was inappropriate (26). A study of cognitively intact patients over age 65 years found that 95% would not desire tube feedings if they were severely demented (27). The issues related to tube feeding of the demented patient have been discussed in detail (28,29).

The Ethics and Humanities Subcommittee of the American Academy of Neurology addressed the issue of feeding tubes in patients with advanced dementia. "Oral hydration and nutrition are offered, assisted and encouraged, but hydration and nutrition are not provided by artificial enteral or parenteral means unless they contribute to patient comfort or are chosen by the patient or proxy" (30).

Some family surrogate decision-makers still demand that severely demented patients receive acute care hospitalization and even cardiopulmonary resuscitation and other aggressive, generally unwarranted interventions. The primary care physician can serve a crucial role in providing insight and education for family members regarding these important issues.

Parkinson's Disease

Parkinson's disease affects between one and two percent of individuals 60 years and older. The triad of tremor, rigidity and akinesia characterize patients with idiopathic Parkinson's disease (22). The designation *paralysis agitans* has also been used in the past to denote Parkinson's disease. The differential diagnosis of idiopathic Parkinson's disease includes atherosclerotic Parkinson's due to ischemic injury to the brain and medication side effects, usually neuroleptic drugs with anti-dopaminergic properties.

Dementia may be present in patients with long-standing disease. About 25% of parkinsonian patients with dementia may actually have Lewy body disease.

Other symptoms of Parkinson's disease may include hallucinations, delusions, and gait disorder with a risk of falling and fracture. More than 50% of patients with Parkinson's disease have depression, which will respond to pharmacotherapy, including SSRIs and less preferably, tricyclic antidepressants. Electroconvulsive therapy is also effective in improving depression as well as motor function temporarily in patients with Parkinson's disease.

Primary therapy for patients with Parkinson's disease include dopamine precursors such as L-DOPA with decarboxylase inhibitors, dopamine agonists, and least preferably, anti-cholinergic medications. These medications also have the potential to cause significant side effects of confusion, hallucinations, and postural hypotension. They must be carefully titrated, and patients closely monitored for signs and symptoms of drug toxicity.

After a period of 1 to 2 years, many patients become refractory to dopamine precursor therapy. Side effects including the on-off phenomenon and other poorly understood motor side effects occur with significant frequency. Peak-dose dyskinesias may occur, as well as psychotic manifestations including agitation, confusion, delusions, and visual hallucinations secondary to anti-Parkinson's medications.

Palliative and supportive therapy of the patient with advanced Parkinson's disease consists of fine adjustment of one or more anti-Parkinson medications available today. Constipation occurs with significant frequency and patients must be placed on a bowel regimen to reduce the risk of constipation (Chapter 2). With progressive immobilization, patients may eventually reach a bed fast state.

When the disease has advanced to the stage of severe disability, the palliative care needs are similar to those of patients with advanced Alzheimer's disease. Patients typically have immobility, contractures, and dementia along with bowel and bladder incontinence. Hospice care may be beneficial for those with advanced disease.

Stroke

Stroke is acute brain injury caused by arterial occlusion (80% of patients) or by hemorrhage (20%). "Brain attack" has also been used to describe stroke, but the term "cerebrovascular accident" (CVA) does not accurately describe the stroke syndrome.

About 500,000 Americans are affected by stroke annually. Approximately 25% of patients die of the acute event, 10% of the survivors return to normal function, 48% have residual hemiparesis or other symptoms, and 22% are unable to ambulate independently (22).

Causes of hemorrhagic stroke include subarachnoid hemorrhage due to ruptured berry or saccular aneurysm. The greatest incidence of aneurysmal rupture occurs in the fifth through seventh decades. Approximately 85% of ruptured saccular aneurysms occur in the anterior circulation and 15% in the posterior circulation. Grade V subarachnoid hemorrhage is defined by the presence of deep coma, from which the patient usually does not recover. Other causes of intracranial hemorrhage include hypertensive etiologies, usually involving the basal ganglia. These include the putamen, thalamus, and caudate nucleus. The cerebellum and brain stem are involved less frequently, but usually with devastating effects.

Prognosis

Patients with stroke may demonstrate steady improvement in overall functional status, while others may enter a period of extended decline. Following an acute hemorrhagic or ischemic stroke, strong predictors of early mortality have been developed. These include coma extending more than 3 days in duration, or development of the PVS, defined as patient unresponsiveness for at least 90 days.

Additional poor prognostic indicators include coma or obtundation accompanied by severe myoclonus persisting beyond 3 days after an acute hypoxic-ischemic event. Patients who remained comatose on day three and who had any of the following had a 97% mortality within 2 months: (1) abnormal brain stem responses, (2) absent response to verbal stimulation, (3) absent withdrawal response to pain, (4) serum creatinine greater than 1.5 mg/dL, and (5) age greater than 70 years (3).

Additional predictors of early stroke mortality include dysphagia severe enough to compromise oral intake of food or fluids, and CT or MRI changes indicating severe structural brain damage (i.e., brain stem hemorrhage or extensive hemorrhage involving the cerebral hemispheres).

Patients who enter a chronic phase following recovery from acute stroke may have characteristics associated with poor survival. These patients may be candidates for palliative care, and may also be hospice candidates. Risk factors include age greater than 70 years; poor functional status with Karnofsky score of less than 50%; post-stroke dementia as evidenced by a FAST score of greater than 7; poor nutritional status even if provided by artificial means and associated with unintentional progressive weight loss of more than 10% over the previous 6 months; and serum albumin less than 2.5 gm/dL. Serum albumin should not be used independently as a sole prognostic indicator.

Comorbid conditions that adversely affect prognosis and may predict progressive clinical decline include aspiration pneumonia, upper urinary tract infection, sepsis, refractory decubitus ulcers, and recurrent fever despite antibiotic therapy (4,8).

Palliative care

Comfort care for the patient with severe stroke follows the general guidelines used for the support of patients with advanced Alzheimer's disease or other debilitating neurological conditions. This includes pain assessment and treatment and frequent repositioning of the patient in an attempt to prevent pressure sores. The latter preventive measures may not always succeed despite everyone's best efforts.

The issue of nutritional support can be a dilemma. Note the above discussion of tube feeding, as well as the discussion in Chapter 11. Family expectations may be unrealistic at first, but with time the inability of the patient to recover becomes apparent. When it is clear that there will be no recovery, tube feedings can be discontinued at the direction of surrogate decision-makers (26,27). The existence of numerous decision-making dilemmas underscores the need to improve access for multidisciplinary palliative care for nursing home patients (31).

The primary focus should be on maintaining maximal comfort for these patients, while understanding that it will not be possible to maintain optimal nutritional status or to prevent weight loss. Even pressure sores are not always preventable, even under the best conditions in which patients can be provided care.

Locked-in Syndrome

The locked-in syndrome, or de-efferented state, results from damage to the pontine tegmentum. These unfortunate patients are totally paralyzed except for preservation of minimal vertical eye movements and occasional remnants of eye blinking. They are fully conscious and aware of their surroundings, and can respond to the examiner using simple communication mechanisms of vertical eye movements or blinking (3). The locked-in syndrome may be caused by ischemic hypoxic injury to the pons, or may be posttraumatic.

Clinical features of the locked-in syndrome include quadri-plegia, pseudobulbar palsy, as well as paralysis of horizontal eye movements. These patients may be incorrectly diagnosed as being comatose, but are actually fully aware of their surroundings and capable of responding in rudimentary fashion with coded eye movements.

Prognosis and decision-making

Many of these patients die soon after the acute event, but some are capable of living for extended periods of time with aggressive supportive care. The bioethical dilemmas and decision-making issues are similar to those faced by the patient with amyotrophic lateral sclerosis.

A previously completed advance directive or history of expressed wishes to a family surrogate decision-maker is invaluable in guiding therapy and supportive care. In the absence of a clear directive, the physician and family should do what is in the best interest of the patient. The focus should be on maximizing quality of life for the patient whenever possible. If there is no expectation for meaningful quality of life, most of us (as potential patients) would prefer to avoid aggressive life-extending interventions.

Surrogate decision-makers and the physician, with the assistance of the Medical Ethics Committee if necessary, can help arrive at critical decisions. The patient with the locked-in syndrome must be encouraged to participate by communicating with limited eye movements.

The principles of supportive care are similar to those discussed for other disorders of motor function.

Coma

Coma is defined as a state of unresponsiveness in which the patient has eyes closed, and cannot be aroused by auditory or painful stimuli. The comatose patient has no awareness of self or surroundings, and cannot experience pain or other sensory stimuli. Reflex motor movements familiar to the neurologist may occur with application of painful stimuli, but these do not indicate that the patient senses pain. Sleep-wake cycles are absent. This helps distinguish coma from patients with PVS in which sleep-wake cycles are actually preserved. Both clinical and electroencephalogram (EEG) criteria may be useful in making the determination of whether sleep-wake cycles are present.

The etiology of coma includes traumatic and non-traumatic injury. The common causes are stroke, anoxic encephalopathy after cardiac arrest, severe hypoglycema, drug overdose, encephalitis, meningitis, and head trauma.

Prognosis

Coma is either reversible or permanent depending on its etiology and duration. Table 6-1, while not exhaustive, reviews clinical indicators of poor prognosis (3).

TABLE 6-1	*Prognosis with Coma*

Conditions with a poor prognosis that are evident soon after the onset of coma (there is little hope for improvement with prolonged support) (3)

▶ Pontine hemorrhage with hyperthermia and extension to midbrain and thalamus

▶ Multiple hemorrhagic contusions with associated extradural hematoma and brain swelling

▶ Gunshot wounds to the head with intraventricular and intracerebral hemorrhage and disseminated intravascular coagulation

▶ Complete cervical cord transection with apnea

▶ Myoclonus, status epilepticus, and brain swelling after cardiac arrest

▶ Multiple infarcts and brain swelling after cardiac surgery

▶ Basilar artery occlusion

▶ Multiple intracranial hemorrhages associated with use of tissue plasminogen activator

Clinical decision-making, and palliative care

Preferences for end-of-life care may have been expressed in an advance directive if the comatose patient had completed such a document. In the absence of this, family surrogate decision-makers discuss care planning with the physician in a manner that would respect the wishes of the comatose patient if previously expressed.

Ethical dilemmas related to life-prolonging interventions have been reviewed in the discussion of other neurological illnesses (i.e., PEG, mechanical ventilation, and antibiotic therapy). All stakeholders—family and clinicians—should keep in mind that prolonging life in extremely dire circumstances may in fact be prolonging the dying process. Issues confronting patients with severe life-limiting neurological disease illustrate the urgent need to improve end-of-life care (32).

Persistent Vegetative State

The term "persistent vegetative state" (PVS) was first used in 1972 to define a neurological condition associated with eyes-open coma, indicating a state of wakefulness but without awareness (3). The pathophysiology of PVS reflects severe diffuse cerebral cortical damage, as well as injury to thalamic neurons and white matter connections. The brain stem is essentially spared, as are hypothalamic neurons.

Head trauma, massive stroke, and anoxic encephalopathy (usually after prolonged cardiopulmonary arrest) are common causes of PVS. In contrast to true coma, patients with PVS have preserved sleep-wake cycles. Neither patients in coma or PVS have any awareness of surroundings, and are incapable of responding to sensory stimuli, including pain.

The Multi-Society Task Force on PVS defined this condition as a vegetative state lasting longer than one month (33). Criteria developed by the task force are summarized in Table 6-2.

Patients with PVS can blink, move their eyes, swallow, breathe, grimace, vocalize, and even move extremities non-purposefully. Unsustained visual pursuit may be evident for a few seconds. Intact subcortical motor reflexes may be associated with stereotyped motor activity. An estimated 5 to 10,000 patients in PVS are maintained in the US alone, mostly in long-term care facilities (3).

The term "locked-out" syndrome has been applied to patients in PVS, since the cerebral cortex is disconnected from the external world. This is in contrast to patients with the "locked-in syndrome" who demonstrate preserved awareness and capacity to respond even though affected with profound paralysis.

TABLE 6-2	*Diagnostic Criteria for the Persistent Vegetative State (PVS) (3)*

▶ Patients have no awareness of themselves or their environment; they are incapable of interacting with others

▶ There is no evidence of sustained reproducible, purposeful, or voluntary behavior or response to visual, auditory, tactile, or noxious stimuli

▶ There is no language comprehension or expression

▶ Patients exhibit intermittent wakefulness manifested by the presence of sleep-wake cycles

▶ Patients have sufficiently preserved autonomic functions of the hypothalamus and brain stem that enable them to survive for extended periods of time if provided adequate medical and nursing support

▶ There is bowel and bladder incontinence

▶ There is evidence of cranial nerve function, such as pupillary, oculocephalic, corneal, vestibulo-ocular and gag responses, and spinal reflexes

Ethical and clinical decision-making issues and the principles of palliation are similar to those discussed for others with advanced neurological illnesses. There is legal precedent for permitting family surrogate decision-makers to withhold and withdraw life support including artificial nutrition and hydration. Surveys clearly indicate that the majority of the American public would not wish to have their lives prolonged if they were in a state of permanent coma or PVS.

References

1. World Health Organization. Cancer Pain Relief and Palliative Care. WHO Technical Report Series 804. Geneva: World Health Organization, 1990:11.

2. Hospice Care. A physician's guide. 2nd printing. National Hospice and Palliative Care Organization, 2001.

3. Bernat JL. Ethical issues in neurology. 2nd ed. Boston: Butterworth Heinemann, 2002.

4. Carver AC, Foley KM. Palliative care in neurology. Neurol Clin 2001;194:789–1044.

5. Caracini A, Martini C. Neurological Problems. In: Oxford textbook of palliative medicine. 2nd ed. New York: Oxford University Press, 1998:727–749.

6. Voltz R, Borasio GD, Bernat JL, et al, eds. Palliative care in neurology. Contemporary Neurology Series. London: Oxford University Press, 2003 (in press).

7. Voltz R, Borasio GD. Palliative therapy in the terminal stage of neurologic disease. J of Neurology 1997;244:S2–S10.

8. Doyle D, Hanks GWC, MacDonald N, eds. Oxford textbook of palliative medicine. 2nd ed. New York: Oxford University Press, 1998.

9. Borasio GD, Walsh D, eds. Palliative care in amyotrophic lateral sclerosis. Motor neuron disease. London: Oxford University Press, 2000.

10. Borasio GD, Voltz R. Palliative care in amyotrophic lateral sclerosis. J Neurology 1997;244:S11–S17.

11. Mitsumoto H, Chad DA, Pioro EP. Amyotrophic lateral sclerosis. Philadelphia: FA Davis Company, 1998.

12. Johnston M, Earll L, Mitchell E, et al. Communicating the diagnosis of motor neuron disease. Pall Med 1996;10:23–34.

13. Buckman R. How to break bad news. London: Papermac, 1996.

14. Oliver D, Borasio GD, Walsh D, eds. Palliative care in amyotrophic lateral sclerosis. Motor neuron disease. London: Oxford University Press, 2000.

15. Lo B, Ruston D, Kates LW, et al. Discussing religious and spiritual issues at the end of life. A practical guide for physicians. JAMA 2002;287:749–754.

16. Irish DP, Lundquist KF, Nelsen VJ, eds. Ethnic variations in dying, death, and grief. Diversity in universality. Philadelphia: Taylor and Francis, 1993.

17. Hopp FP, Duffy SA. Racial variations in end-of-life care. JAGS, 2000;48:658–663.

18. Crawley LV, Payne R, Bolden J, et al. Palliative and end-of-life care in the African American community. JAMA 2000;284:2518–2521.

19. Lacomblez L, Bensimon G, Leigh PN, et al. Dose-ranging study of riluzole in amyotrophic lateral sclerosis. Lancet 1996;347:1425–1431.

20. Aboussouan LS, Khan SU, Meeker DP, et al. Effect of non-invasive positive pressure ventilation on survival in amyotrophic lateral sclerosis. Ann of Int Med 1997;127:450–453.

21. Mulder DW, ed. The diagnosis and treatment of amyotrophic lateral sclerosis. Boston: Houghton Mifflin, 1980.

22. Samuels MA, ed. Manual of neurologic therapeutics. 6th ed. Philadelphia: Lippincott Williams and Wilkins, 1999.

23. Carney MT, Neugroschl J, Morrison RS, et al. The development and piloting of a capacity assessment tool. J Clin Ethics 2001;12:17–23.

24. Howe EG. How to determine competency. J Clin Ethics 2001;12:3–16.

25. Management of cancer pain. Clinical practice guideline: US Dept. of Health and Human Services, Agency for Health Care Policy and Research. Publication #94-0592, March 1994.

26. Hodges MO, Tolle SW, Stocking C, Cassel CK. Tube feeding: internists' attitudes regarding ethical obligations. Arch Intern Med 1994;154: 1013–1020.

27. Gjerdingen DK, Neff JA, Wang M, et al. Older persons' opinions about life-sustaining procedures in the face of dementia. Arch Fam Med 1999;8:421–425.

28. Gillick MR. Rethinking the role of tube feeding in patients with advanced dementia. N Engl J Med 2000;342:206–210.

29. Gillick MR. Artificial nutrition and hydration in the patient with advanced dementia: is withholding treatment compatible with traditional Judaism? J Med Ethics 2001;27:12–15.

30. American Academy of Neurology Ethics and Humanities Subcommittee. Ethical issues in the management of the demented patient. Neurology 1996;46:1180–1183.

31. Zerzan J, Stearns S, Hanson L. Access to palliative care and hospice in nursing homes. JAMA 2000;284:2489–2494.

32. A controlled trial to improve care for seriously ill hospitalized patients. The Study to Understand Prognosis and Preferences for Outcomes and Risks of Treatments (SUPPORT). JAMA 1995;274:1591–1598.

33. Multi-Society Task Force on PVS. Medical aspects of the persistent vegetative state. N Engl J Med 1994;330:1499–1508.

7 | AIDS

Harlee S. Kutzen

There is no cure for HIV infection. With continued treatment we hope to suppress viral replication for as long as possible while simultaneously attempting to prevent life threatening opportunistic infection (OI). But ultimately, all who have AIDS need palliative, supportive treatment. HIV is not like other diseases of our time. It is communicable, stigmatized, expensive to treat, and affects millions of citizens of the world. HIV disproportionately kills the most vulnerable among us: the impoverished, uneducated, mentally ill, homeless, substance users, and prisoners. These communities may be hard to reach, and they generally have little political power and few advocates.

Advance care planning and end-of-life HIV care is complex. Every member of the HIV care team should understand how HIV affects each patient and family. They must adjust to the issues of stigma, isolation, secrecy, disease disclosure, anger, guilt, and sadness in the face of premature death. Their tasks include blending highly active antiretroviral therapies (HAART) with palliative care, and treating the complex medical conditions associated with advanced HIV. In addition to these technical aspects of medical care, they must deal with the psychosocial issues unique to HIV, and also work with community resources for care and support (1–4).

Unique aspects of HIV palliative care

There are many aspects of palliative care that are unique to individuals, families, and communities affected by HIV disease (Table 7-1). The availability of new antiretroviral agents and the rapid evolution of new information has introduced extraordinary complexity into the treatment of HIV-infected persons. New therapies that reduce HIV viral load work best for patients able to tolerate side effects and for those who can afford them and have social support.

New therapies have increased survival for persons with HIV and AIDS, and have given them more symptom-free years (5). On

TABLE 7-1	*Unique Aspects of HIV Palliative Care*

- Relative youth of patients
- Infected families (including mother, father, and children)
- Complexity of HIV disease
- Rapidly changing knowledge base
- Unpredictable response to therapy
- Complex issues of hope
- Marginalized communities (African Americans, Hispanics/Latinos, mentally ill, women, substance users, and prisoners) disproportionately affected
- Skyrocketing costs of HIV antiretrovirals
- Many of the same medications used to treat the HIV virus are used for prophylaxis and palliation
- Chronicity of conditions reduces observation of "signals" of advancing disease
- Legal issues regarding HIV disclosure
- Whole family infections—HIV infected partners, parents and children, and transmission guilt
- Management of complex pain symptoms more challenging with active substance users (and family members)

- Roller coaster course of disease causes loss of prognosis predictors
- Isolated mourners due to secret loved one's HIV status
- Contagion, fear of fatal infection
- Multiple losses within communities related to death (there are more orphans)
- Spouses, partners, and caregivers often HIV-infected—facing their own future care needs and deaths
- Postponed guardianship for children due to denial of approaching death
- Stigma
- Isolation
- Many common non-HIV cofactors complicate care in high percent of care population (substance abuse, poverty, mental illness, hepatitis C, HTLV I, homelessness, cardiovascular disease)
- Health community frequently denies death and advancing disease in the era of "high hopes" for viral suppression
- Patients die unexpectedly (other medical conditions, sepsis, homicide, suicide)

the other hand, we cannot discount the complications associated with HAART and the compromises patients and families make in their attempts to adhere to complex regimens of HAART, OI prophylaxis, and palliative care medications and treatments (Table 7-2). Treatment strategies are continuously evolving, and a thorough review of them is beyond our purpose. The most current information about treatment is readily available via numerous Internet resources (Box 7-1).

TABLE 7-2	*Complications of Highly Active Antiretroviral Therapies (HAART)*

▶ High pill burden (some patients are taking 70–100 pills/d combining palliative medications + HAART)	▶ "Lazarus-like" syndrome (appearing close to death, and unexpectedly improving greatly)
▶ Dietary complications—some medications with food, some without, some with high acidic food, others not	▶ Roller coaster adjustments of good days and bad
▶ Numerous severe side effects	▶ Increased cardiovascular risks
▶ Drug resistance/Failing regimens	▶ Liver and renal toxicities
▶ Clinically contradictory states—patients who feel & look horrible, yet have great viral/immune markers & vice versa	▶ Adherence challenges
	▶ Impaired quality of life
	▶ Changing aspects of hope (hoping for viral suppression and long life, then eventually hoping for quality of life and support at end of life

BOX 7-1	*HIV clinical care and treatment guidelines via Internet resources*

http://www.aids.org/

http://www.ama-assn.org/special/hiv/

http://www.cdcnpin.org/

http://www.fda.gov/oashi/aids/hiv.html

http://sis.nlm.nih.gov/hiv.cfm

http://www.actis.org/

http://www.aegis.com/

http://www.hopkins-aids.edu/

http://www.hsph.harvard.edu/organizations/hai/

http://www.pedhivaids.org/

Blending HAART and Palliative Care

When do our efforts shift from trying to save the patient to palliation and end-of-life care? Often there is no discernible shift. It may seem a paradox, but it is common for HIV care providers to simultaneously plan for advanced disease and death amidst a flurry of activity to control the HIV virus. They may not get it right; in practice, emphasis may be on aggressive antiretroviral therapies even when the HIV-infected person is emaciated, profoundly weak, repeatedly hospitalized, and has no interest in further diagnostic testing.

Furthermore, we frequently encounter individuals who are not only at the end of their lives, but who do not know they are HIV-infected and are dying of HIV-related conditions. Such patients can be difficult to care for when we do not know whether to begin aggressive therapies or refer to hospice. This can be a point of conflict for HIV interdisciplinary care teams.

Advances in HIV treatment have complicated the determination of what exactly "advanced HIV" looks like, and they have blurred the edges of HIV palliative care (5,6). For these reasons, it is difficult to distinguish when HIV care is specifically treatment-focused and when it is exclusively palliative. Now we generally refer to advanced HIV care as a blending of HAART and palliative care. HAART therapy is ordered not only for aggressive treatment of HIV viral load suppression, but also to reduce some of the uncomfortable symptoms of viremia even when complete suppression is not achieved.

Some effects of increased survival—We have seen the paradoxical condition of individuals with the most advanced stages of disease prepare for the end of their life only to find that a new medication combination has improved their health and immune status (a Lazarus-like syndrome). We have also seen individuals who have outlived all of their friends, family members, and support systems, bearing witness to incredible loss and suffering, living with fears for their own support when they are at the end of their lives.

Increasing longevity with advanced HIV increases the potential for more neurological deficits. Individuals are living longer with dementia, altered gait, poor proprioception, and increasing safety concerns. Providers struggle with ethical issues of whether or not to support renewal of an individual's motor vehicle license, or whether or not an individual can safely return home after an extended hospital stay and mental deterioration. Other common issues include:

▶ There is an increased incidence of hepatitis C (HCV) coinfection which influences advanced care planning for those with HIV. Inability to tolerate hepatotoxic medications and liver failure increase morbidity and mortality.

▶ Active substance abuse compounds morbidity and mortality with advancing HIV because of a general failure of self-care, continued engagement in high risk activities, and increased risk of exposure to additional drug resistant strains of HIV.

▶ There are more people with difficulty accessing and negotiating systems of health care who need special support.

Prognosis

Prognosis is more difficult to define with AIDS than it is with malignancy, or even with advanced heart or lung disease. One difficulty is that HIV has a variable course of illness studded with plateaus. Another is the occasionally surprising effect of a new therapy on people with advanced disease. Review of the HIV websites and journals indicates an overwhelming emphasis on disease treatment over projections of life expectancy. Table 7-3 and Box 7-2 provide a general framework for deciding that a patient has limited survival (5–7).

TABLE 7-3	*Frequently Encountered Complications of Advanced HIV Infection Requiring Specific Therapy*
Affected System	**Diagnoses (this list is not complete)**
Brain/CNS	Lymphoma, cryptococcal meningitis, toxoplasmosis, neurosyphilis, HIV dementia, seizures
Systemic infections	Multiple protozoal, bacterial, fungal, and viral infections rarely encountered in those with a competent immune system
Respiratory	*Pneumocystis* pneumonia, tuberculosis, histoplasmosis, and other fungal infections, Kaposi's sarcoma of the lung, sinusitis
Malignancies	Non-Hodgkin lymphoma, Kaposi's sarcoma of lungs or gastrointestinal tract, cervical cancer (papilloma virus-associated)
Gastrointestinal	Thrush, HIV enteropathy with diarrhea and malabsorption, infectious diarrhea, rectal lesions
Skin	Seborrheic dermatitis, folliculitis, shingles (and other skin infections)
Others	Liver or renal disease, chronic pancreatitis (often drug related); cardiomyopathy, active substance abuse

| BOX 7-2 | *Criteria for HIV-related hospice referral* |

▶ When patients have failed available therapeutic antiretroviral therapies

▶ Demonstration of inability to tolerate HAART with advanced disease

▶ Continuing on expanded access medication regimens for chronic symptom management only

▶ Impaired quality of life due to advanced HIV symptoms

▶ Patient and/or family express distress regarding end-of-life issues

▶ Diagnosis of life-limiting AIDS-related condition such as CNS non-Hodgkin's lymphoma, recurrent/resistant co-infections, and/or end-stage organ failure

▶ Expression of feeling tired after years of complex medication/ treatment regimens, failing therapies, and desiring a simpler, higher quality of life

▶ When after-hour on-call needs for symptom management or support exceed the capacities that of the outpatient clinic and emergency room

Laboratory evaluation may help establish prognosis. When the CD4+ T cell count falls below 200 cells per microliter there is increased risk of OI, but with HAART and prophylaxis against the common OIs such as *Pneumoncystis carinii* patients can live for years. When the cell count is below 50 per microliter AIDS is considered end-stage, and those with counts below 10 usually die within a year. The viral load is an independent indicator of disease severity, and it should decline with HAART. Those not receiving HAART and who have high levels of serum HIV-1 RNA, or who continue to have high viral titers despite antiviral therapy have a poor prognosis.

Prognosis is determined by a complex mix of general health status, OIs, the blend of prophylaxis and treatment strategies and whether or not there is central nervous system (CNS) involvement. AIDS related dementia tends to be progressive, and when advanced indicates limited survival. Many surrogate decision-making and clinicians elect to stop HAART when dementia is severe. That is often the case with AIDS-related malignancy as well.

Many of our patients will not receive HAART, for a variety of reasons. Those in marginalized groups (e.g., the homeless, mentally ill, and drug abusers) come to treatment late, and often are unable to comply with the difficult treatment regimen. In the absence of HAART and/or prophylaxis for OI, prognosis is more easily determined by laboratory findings and clinical status.

HIV-related inpatient hospital admission is frequently a marker of advancing HIV disease. Multiple admissions within a year usually indicate poor short-term prognosis, and also indicate a need for increased support and palliative care services. This should not be postponed until the patient is terminal.

When and how to refer to hospice

Because patients and health care providers may never reach the point of relinquishing aggressive therapies until just before death, we must expand our view of palliative care. There has to be a blend; we do not stop aggressive treatment and start palliation (an approach that may describe treatment of some cancers). For patients who are continuing to progress in their HIV disease, or have life limiting comorbidities (Table 7-3) we must consider 100% palliative care. Box 7-2 describes critical factors to consider before referring to hospice.

Discussing palliative care with the patient and family—In our society, hospice care is often perceived as giving up curative treatment and getting ready to die. As is often the case in medicine, the effective caregiver begins a discussion by listening. Ask the patient and family what they are currently doing with support services, and what hospice care means to them. It usually works better if you are sitting close to the patient and at eye level. Box 7-3 provides openings and questions that will help guide your discussion. The conversation usually does not happen in one setting, but over a series of visits. If you present the "argument for palliative care" in one breath and require a decision, the decision will probably be "no." The patient needs time to digest this information, and to discuss it with family and friends. It is especially useful to have the patient's caregiver and surrogate decision-maker participate in some of the discussion.

People living with HIV commonly defer hospice until late in their life. In fact, many never accept hospice care, even when you consider it the best option, and even when you have done your

BOX 7-3	*Entrees into discussion of end-of-life planning*

What has your medical provider told you about your condition? What does this information mean to you?

Tell me about your good days . . . what are you able to do on those days?

When is the last time you had a day like that in the past 2 months?

What kind of assistance do you need on days when you do not feel well?

If your condition worsens, do you wish to go to the hospital? What do you expect they will do for you there?

Do you have advance directives, such as a living will or durable power of attorney for health care? Who in your family is aware of this and has copies?

Have you discussed treatment preferences with your durable power of attorney for health care? Are they in agreement with your preferences and desires if you are no longer able to speak for yourself? If this person is not a member of your family, do your relatives understand that he or she will be your surrogate decision-maker?

In the event of your condition getting worse, is there anyone you are worried about in the event of your death (children, spouse, partner, friends, parents, pets, etc.)?

Are you having any pain or distressing symptoms now? In what ways are they impairing the quality of your life and your ability to accomplish important goals/activities?

What are the most important components of your life at this time?

What can we do to make your life more comfortable?

best to explain it. Box 7-4 addresses common reasons for delayed referral to hospice and strategies to facilitate acceptance of such referrals. It is helpful to point out that hospice can be considered particularly effective home health care, incorporating a higher level of clinical expertise, on-call availability and other special support services (Chapter 1).

But in the end, we must remember that hospice is the patient's choice, and it will be refused by some who perceive hospice as "giving up hope."

| BOX 7-4 | *Reasons for delayed hospice referral for HIV-infected patients* |

▶ Lack of a consensus among the members on the determination of end-stage status

▶ Patient/family misunderstanding of hospice concept—believe they must relinquish all medications, including those which prevent infections and keep them comfortable

▶ Patients strive to live for the day when the "cure" is found

▶ Some disenfranchised or minority families feel if they do not have ongoing aggressive life-saving measures available their care will be sub-standard (see Chapter 1)

▶ Patients and providers hope for positive response in the next set of new and untried antiretroviral therapies

▶ Many women with young children fear that signing up for hospice care may cause them to die sooner than they want in order to accomplish important end-of-life tasks

▶ There are unexpected deaths associated with severe sepsis, unspecified causes, homicides, and suicides

▶ No matter how you word it, hospice care represents end-of-life care

Ways to Facilitate Acceptance of Hospice by HIV-infected Patients

▶ Evaluate the degree to which you have educated the patient/family about home support options

▶ Emphasize that hospice is similar to other home health care service, but with more sophisticated resources (skillful nurses able to administer medicines and draw blood for laboratory work, on-call coverage, etc.)

▶ Give the patient and family the freedom to choose hospice

▶ Write out a prescription for hospice, reminding patients of their trust in the previous care offered and how we are still just as invested in their best interest as ever

▶ Let the patient know if their care improves, and they no longer need or desire hospice care, they may be discharged

▶ For patients who express concerns about loved ones, they may take great comfort in learning about the year of hospice bereavement follow-up support after their death

HIV symptom management

Table 7-4 reviews symptoms associated with advanced HIV and HAART that diminish quality of life and necessitate palliation. HIV symptom management simultaneously addresses viral suppression, opportunistic infection treatment and prevention, side effects of medications, pre-existing medical conditions, and other social and physical needs (8,9).

Pain is noted across the entire spectrum of HIV disease (10,11). Particular pains associated with advanced HIV include peripheral neuropathy, bone and joint, visceral, and frequently procedural pain. The principles of pain management outlined in Chapter 2 apply.

There is increasing evidence of both weight loss and malnutrition as HIV disease progresses. Changes in body

TABLE 7-4	*Complications of Therapy and Advanced AIDS/HIV Disease*

Symptoms Associated with HAART	Symptoms Associated with Advanced HIV
▶ Nausea/vomiting	▶ Nausea
▶ Diarrhea	▶ Diarrhea or constipation
▶ Insomnia	▶ Changes in sleep patterns
▶ Nightmares	▶ Skin changes and/or oral changes
▶ Dizziness	▶ Anemia
▶ Headaches	▶ Increasing fatigue/weakness
▶ Joint and muscle aches	▶ Anorexia/cachexia
▶ Elevated triglycerides	▶ Neuromuscular and neurological changes
▶ Lipodystrophy	▶ Pain—multiple sites/different sources
▶ Rashes	including peripheral neuropathies; joint and muscle aches
▶ Anemia	▶ Fevers
▶ Fatigue	▶ Seizures
▶ Peripheral neuropathies	▶ Nightsweats
▶ Weight loss	▶ Vision loss
▶ Dry mouth	▶ Hiccups
▶ Pancreatitis	▶ Mental status changes
▶ Hepatitis	▶ Anxiety/depression
	▶ Dyspnea

composition, body image perception, digestion, tolerance of food intake, and side effects of therapies add to a reduced quality of life. Even when patients have adequate food, nutrition knowledge, resources and support, they may be unable to maintain weight. Consultation with a dietician who has experience treating patients with AIDS may help.

As the patient gets weaker, symptom management becomes entirely dependent on their lay caregivers. Caregivers need special help and specific instructions about pain and symptom management. They should be included when establishing and agreeing on the overall goals of care, the likelihood of symptoms, how to access support and guidance, and a plan for end-of-life care.

Community aspects of HIV care

Society, and particularly the health care community, is so enticed by visions of an AIDS cure that it exhibits signs of denial about death from AIDS. Sadly, death from AIDS is a fact of life, and AIDS will continue to be a leading killer of young people. For this reason, we must temper our desire to "overcome death" with realistic planning for end-of-life care.

AIDS will be with us for the foreseeable future. Unfortunately, we must plan for the infection of whole families and communities. We cannot ignore marginalized groups with special needs: substance abusers, the mentally ill, and the homeless to name a few. In the face of sky-rocketing costs of life-long antiviral treatment, we must strategically build palliative care into the spectrum of HIV care, education, and life planning.

References

1. Aronstein DM, Thompson BJ, eds. HIV and social work: a practitioner's guide. New York: Harrington Parker Press, 1998.
2. Corless IB, Nicholas PK. Long-term continuum of care for people living with HIV/AIDS. J Urban Health 2000;77:176–186.
3. Ferris F, Flannery J, eds. A comprehensive guide for the care of persons with HIV disease: module 4: palliative care. Toronto: Mount Sinai Hospital/Casey Hospice, 1995.
4. Greenburg B, McCorkle R, Vlahov D, Selwyn PA. Palliative care for HIV disease in the era of highly active antiretroviral therapy. Bulletin of the New York Academy of Medicine. J Urban Health 2000;77:150–165.
5. Dore GJ, Li Y, McDonald A, et al. Impact of highly active antiretroviral therapy on individual defining illness incidence and survival in Australia. J Acquired Immune Defic Syndrome 2002;29:388–395.

6. Lundgren JD, Mocoft A, Gatell JM, et al. A clinically prognositic scoring system for patients receiving highly active antiretroviral therapy results from the EuroSIDA study. J Infect Dis 2002;185:178–187.

7. Vergis EN, Mellors JW. Natural history of HIV-1 infection. Infect Dis Clin of North Am 2000;14:809–825.

8. Armes PJ, Higginson IJ. What constitutes high-quality HIV/AIDS palliative care. J Palliat Care 1999;15:5–12.

9. Alexander C. Palliative care and end-of-life care. A guide to the clinical care of women with HIV. U.S. Department of Health and Human Services, Health Resources and Services Administration, HIV/AIDS Bureau, 2001:343–376.

10. Newshan G, Sherman DW. Palliative care: pain and symptom management in persons with HIV/AIDS. Nurs Clin North Am 1999;34:131–134.

11. Holzemer WL, Henry SB, Reilly CA. Assessing and managing pain in AIDS care: the patient perspective. J Assoc Nurses AIDS Care 1998;9:22–30.

8 Cancer

Frank J. Brescia

The cancer burden to our society and health care system remains formidable (1). The estimated number of newly diagnosed patients with cancer in the United States for 2002 is approximately 1,300,000. Breast, prostate, lung, and colorectal malignancies will account for 55% of all cancers, with prostate and breast cancers contributing nearly one-third of new cases. Cancer causes about one-fourth of deaths in the United States, and is the second leading cause of death after cardiovascular disease. It is the leading cause of death among women aged 40 to 79, and among men aged 60 to 79. After accidents, it is the second leading cause of death in children under age 15. Lung, prostate, breast, and colon cancer account for more than half of the cancer deaths.

Despite advances in the understanding of cancer biology, epidemiology, and treatment, nearly half the patients diagnosed eventually die from their disease (1). The majority of patients with advanced solid tumors (e.g., extensive local or metastatic disease) will eventually require palliative care, and fewer than 10% of them are cured with currently available therapy.

When cancer is detected in its early stage and cure is the goal, severe side effects of a possibly successful therapy may seem acceptable to many patients. On the other hand, advanced malignancies rarely have complete tumor response to therapy, and even when clinical remissions occur, the effect on survival remains modest or negligible. At this stage of illness the calculation of risk (toxicity) versus benefits of treatment is more important, and must be clearly explained to the patient. All concerned—patient, family, and doctor—should realistically face what is to likely happen and not what they hope will happen. If treatment designed to prolong life is certain to fail, then all measures should be directed at *just* symptom control.

This, of course, presupposes that the medical oncologist can recognize when anti-tumor therapies will no longer work. In practice, that point in time can be hard to define. Even though it is imprecise, there comes a time in the course of every illness when it is apparent that treatment is not working and the terminal phase of the illness has begun. Palliation, other end-of-life support measures, and a peaceful death become the goals of care. The response of the clinician at this time fundamentally affects the final experience of the patient.

Phases of cancer treatment

Barriers to effective end-of-life care are discussed in Chapter 1. Patients with cancer and their families often refuse to accept a plan that does not include antitumor therapy. They may be unrealistic about the risks or toxicities of therapy. They may be concerned that the doctor will lose interest when there is no longer an attempt to cure the disease, as our health care culture— including oncology—is preoccupied with cure. For these and other reasons, one study found that 53% of patients were willing to accept chemotherapy with all its toxicity for a 1% chance of cure! Forty percent would accept intensive therapy that would extend their lives by only 3 months (2).

For a typical patient with cancer, there usually are discrete decision points: at the time of diagnosis, during remission and surveillance, at the time of recurrence, during second or third-line treatment, during salvage treatment, and finally, with hospice care at end of life (last days). There has been limited research regarding the range of patient choices and needs during these different phases. Bruera found that the doctor and patient agreed on the stage of illness and prognosis in less than half the cases (in addition to uncertainty there are substantial problems with communication). As one might anticipate, the majority of patients (63%) preferred and expected that there would be agreement with their doctor (3).

Acceptance that no treatment will or can be directed against the tumor may vary among patients and family members, often creating conflict and tension. When the physician continues to recommend more anti-cancer treatments while the patient recognizes that therapy will not help and has accepted that death is approaching, there may be a mix of confusion, anger, and even guilt (at "giving up"). These conflicts make a person's last months or days more difficult.

Clinical decisions

The ability to relieve the complex problems of advanced cancer begins with an understanding of tumor behavior and pathophysiology. When a patient with cancer develops new symptoms, the usual cause is the cancer, itself. Thus, reducing the tumor burden often relieves symptoms. A knowledge of both the natural history of a specific cancer (what it will or will not do), as well as the tempo of progression, allows the clinician to anticipate and manage the changing picture of illness. Box 8-1 provides general principles that help with clinical decision-making when there is extensive disease. At this time there may be confusion and uncertainty, and there are questions that must be answered by a competent oncologist. For you, the patient's primary care doctor, it is useful to understand the big picture, and to know what questions to ask.

Predicting survival and prognosis

Even experienced oncologists have difficulty accurately predicting the life expectancy of a patient with advanced cancer. Uncertainty is hard on patients and families. Furthermore, Medicare requires identifying a 6-month prognosis as eligibility for hospice benefits. Better estimates of prognosis would also help clinical decision-making including the selection of patients for palliation rather than aggressive therapy.

Christakis evaluated the survival of Medicare patients after they had been enrolled in hospice programs (4). Using 1990 Medicare claims data, he analyzed the survival of 6451 hospice patients. The median survival after enrollment was 36 days with 16% of the patients dying within 7 days of hospice admission, while almost 15% survived longer than 6 months. Survival was shortest for renal failure, leukemia, lymphoma, and liver or biliary cancer, and it tended to be longer with dementia, chronic lung disease, and breast cancer. With just 36-day survival, most of these patients were placed into hospice programs late in the course of their illness. At an earlier time survival in hospice was longer, indicating a change in referral patterns.

Few studies have examined our ability to identify the end of life. Llobera found that oncologists were only accurate in 25% of cases (e.g., with their assessment of longevity close enough to be of practical use for the patient and family) (5). Both quality of life parameters (exercise tolerance, weight loss, and activity level) and the stage of disease help establish prognosis (6).

A large study of 1107 advanced cancer patients admitted for terminal care identified eight diverse variables that significantly predicted the risk of dying while in hospital (Table 8-1) (7). It is important to understand the implications of multivariable analysis

| BOX 8-1 | *General principles: Clinical decision making in patients with advanced cancer nearing end of life* |

1. Establish that the cancer is beyond meaningful therapeutic intervention. Patients with treatable tumors should not have just palliative care, unless that is their informed choice. Many with advanced tumors still may be responsive to anti-tumor therapies that improve survival and symptoms (particularly lymphoma, breast, and prostate cancer).

2. Evaluate the relationship between the etiology of the patient's symptoms and the malignancy. Once patients are classified as terminal, inexperienced physicians often assume that tumor reduction is of no benefit. However, in many situations tumor size may be reduced with few side effects, leading to a marked improvement in symptoms.

3. Be sure the patient's symptoms are compatible with the natural history of the particular cancer. For example, it is common for both breast and prostate cancer to metastasize to bone, but this is not as common with other tumors such as ovarian, cervix, or pancreas cancer. In such cases, it would be important to exclude other causes of bone pain (i.e., another cancer, the cancer treatment, polypharmacy, concurrent illness made worse by cancer treatment, emotional issues, or simply another unrelated illness like arthritis).

4. Limit diagnostic studies to those that are absolutely necessary for a patient to gain real benefit. If the information gathered will not meaningfully change the outcome the test should not be done. We should never add to the patient's burden unnecessarily. An obvious rule is not to make things worse, and to follow the Hippocratic "do no harm" mandate.

5. Decide where the patient is located on the trajectory of illness. How close do you think the patient is to death? How surprised would you be if the patient lived 1 month, 3 months, 6 months, 1 year? How rapidly has deterioration occurred (e.g., weight loss or mental status changes, decline in activity tolerance)?

6. Be aware of what important information needs to be communicated and to whom—patient, family, friends, staff.

Continued

How much of what is said is heard, and more importantly, understood? What emotional and cognitive elements are driving decisions—guilt, fear, denial, ambivalence, unrealistic expectations, poor insight, inadequate understanding? How good is the other health care staff in breaking bad news?

7. Define realistic treatment goals. One must examine the personal meaning of futility with the patient and family, but define it with specific objectives—life expectancy, function, pain, satisfaction, quality-of-life, costs. Can we understand the meaning of suffering for any particular individual?

8. Consider how you will respond if the patient and family choose "unconventional options" including alternative care, unproven medicines and obvious quackery? Will the clinical team still care for them?

| TABLE 8-1 | *Risk Factors for Early Mortality in Patients with Cancer** |

---

1. Serum albumin level <2.6 g/dL
2. Lung cancer (either cell type)
3. Lung metastasis
4. Liver metastasis
5. Age 55 to 64 years
6. Depressed socioeconomic status

---

* Multivariate analysis of 1107 patients admitted to hospital with cancer; these variables were independent predictors of death during that hospitalization (7). The nature of multivariable analysis selects the variable that is the strongest predictor. That is to say, cachexia and general debility or mental status changes are certainly predictors of early death, but depressed albumin is found in the same patients, and the analysis found that low albumin was the stronger (and therefore significant) predictor.

---

in this study, and to realize that its goal was to identify the person on the brink of death (not one who would die in 2 to 3 months). Nevertheless, the data help with determining prognosis as a person with two or three of these features is unlikely to live 3 months (and would be a candidate for hospice care). While the multivariable analysis selected low albumin as the significant constitutional predictor of early death, clinical experience indicates that advanced cachexia, severe exercise intolerance, altered mental status, brain metastasis, and other metabolic disorders (i.e., hypercalcemia or hypocholesterolemia) also increase the chance of death within 3 to 6 months.

Doctors tend to err on the side of optimism. A prospective study of survival estimates for 468 terminally ill patients involving 343 clinicians found that only 20% of the doctors were accurate, and 63% were overly-optimistic in their predictions of survival (8). The authors speculated that this error could adversely affect the quality of care of these patients. Often, a patient is stable for prolonged periods with little obvious progression of symptoms. When this is the case, the doctor may be reluctant to take away "hope" and therefore continues active treatment.

It is one thing for the doctor to be wrong when estimating survival. Much worse, and controversial, is when the doctor knowingly misleads about the prognosis and gives the patient false hope. A common reason for this is that some doctors are uncomfortable giving any bad news. Another is the belief that optimistic reports help patients do better clinically, and bad news hastens the progress of the illness (8,9). When interviewed, oncologists have agreed that a "positive attitude" affects outcome of both early and late stage malignancies (9).

I would argue that there are problems with false optimism, regardless of the physician's motives. An inaccurate prognosis may delay the patient's entering an appropriate care program like hospice, thus missing needed services. Another consequence is that the patient may recognize the lie (doctors naively understimate patients' insights). This magnifies feelings of isolation and sets the stage for mistrust. Finally, giving inaccurate information to a patient violates the principle of truth telling (Chapter 1). When asking you a question, a competent person has the right to the most accurate answer you can provide.

Communicating bad new

The patient usually asks, "How much time do I have?" No one answer fits all situations. It is your duty to respond as honestly as possible, relying on what is known about the natural history of the disease. At the same time, you can point out the inherent inaccuracy of prognosis estimates. The need for information must be balanced with the uncertainties.

The effective clinician also uses this opportunity to open a broader discussion of why the question is meaningful for the patient. What is going on in the person's life is relevant. Patients often have specific goals, like wanting to live to witness an important family event (i.e., the birth of a grandchild, a daughter's college graduation, etc.). There may be unfinished family business including reconciliations or resolution of conflicts. The physician and the rest of the health care team do a better job when aware of needs like these, and they are frequent topics of discussion when the hospice team meets.

As noted in Chapter 1, discussions about prognosis and goals often take place over the course of multiple visits, and it is helpful when they include the family. Although the primary care doctor knows the patient well, and is thus in a good position to provide council, the oncologist is usually brought into the discussion to provide information about the natural history of the disease. The general principles of communication outlined in Chapter 1 apply.

With cancer patients it is especially important to state the doctor's ongoing commitment and to address any sense of isolation. Be aware that many patients fear abandonment when there is a diagnosis of cancer. Treatment guidelines, recently adopted for advanced lung cancer by the American Society of Clinical Oncology, are helpful to the practicing clinician (10).

Clinical trials

Large oncology practices, and certainly those in academic centers, participate in multicenter clinical trials and offer experimental therapy when conventional treatment has failed or will not work. Patients agree to enter investigational trials primarily for one reason, to get better. It is worth noting that Phase I studies of investigational drugs offer little chance for success for a person with advanced malignancy; there is a 5% response rate for those who have failed conventional therapy (11).

It is a potentially coercive situation. The desperate patient hopes to get better, and the physician both overestimates the chance for survival and is afraid to deny hope. With this combination it is almost inevitable that the patient gets treated. Many of these therapies have substantial toxicity, and a reasonable assessment of risk versus benefit would favor avoiding treatment. There may be the additional ethical dilemma of the physician-investigator who has a vested interest in enrolling patients in the study, yet is supposed to be the patient's agent (a situation that suggests an important role for the primary care doctor).

This is not an argument against clinical trials, but instead is a suggestion that you pay careful attention to patient selection.

Those with good exercise tolerance, who are still active and who have had little weight loss may be good candidates for clinical trials despite their having incurable cancer. On the other hand, a patient with multiple risk factors for early mortality possibly should avoid them (Table 8-1). Finally, we must all carefully examine the informed consent process for these vulnerable patients.

Symptom Control

Chapter 2 reviews the pharmacology of symptom control, and provides useful general principles of pain management.

Chronic cancer pain

Pain occurs in more than 80% of those with advanced cancer. It is also the most treatable of cancer symptoms, and can be relieved and/or controlled in more than 90% of patients. Nevertheless, most people consider cancer extremely painful, and many avoid seeking treatment because of a belief that therapy will be painful. More alarming is the realization that a substantial number of dying patients do so while experiencing pain that could be controlled, but is not. Cleeland reported that 67% of outpatients with metastatic cancer (871/1305) had pain, and 42% were not receiving adequate analgesic treatment (12). Another study reported that 44% of 101 in-patients at a university hospital had severe pain, and 40% of them had no analgesic order (13). A survey of oncologists reported that a majority of their patients were undermedicated, often because of inadequate pain assessment (14).

Unrelieved pain provokes anxiety and depression, and good management of pain diminishes these emotional problems. On the other hand preexisting depression is not predictive of pain intensity, nor do depressed patients respond less favorably to appropriate pain therapy. The experience of pain is individual and is dependent on more than injury to bodily tissue. *Pain is what the patient says it is.* It is influenced by the psychosocial and even spiritual makeup of an individual, as well as how the person has handled pain in the past.

Early in the course of cancer, pain is less likely to be an issue because it is acute, short-lived, and easily managed. Many times, it is caused by intensive diagnostic or treatment interventions. However, even at this early stage patients can experience severe pain.

With advanced cancer most experience pain that is intense, chronic, progressive, and can be related to a multitude of other complaints (e.g., anorexia, constipation, lethargy, confusion). At this stage of illness, patients are likely to use emotionally charged language to describe their pain: "unbearable," "suffering," "overwhelming."

Pain is most common with solid tumors (i.e., breast, pancreas, prostate, rectum). A study of over 1000 dying patients with cancer identified cervical malignancy as the tumor most associated with severe pain (7). About half of those with documented bone metastasis also report severe pain.

Treatment—The use of analgesics is reviewed in Chapter 2. Cancer pain can be a therapeutic challenge because of the extent of tumor involvement or proximity to nerve structures. Escalation of pain and a need for increasing doses of analgesics usually means worsening of the cancer. Cherny suggests a number of questions when dealing with escalating pain (15).

▶ Are there primary cancer treatments that possibly could help the pain?

▶ Has opioid therapy been maximized to the correct tolerable dose? *The proper dose is the dose that works, and there is no set upper limit.*

▶ Has appropriate adjuvant therapy been considered (steroids, muscle relaxants, anti-seizure or antidepressant medicines, Chapter 2)?

▶ Have side effects been recognized and treated?

▶ Have physical, behavioral, cognitive approaches been best utilized?

Although cancer pain can usually be controlled, the clinician faces a barrage of clinical issues that may complicate treatment (Table 8-2). Non-cancer issues also can create havoc at the bedside: unrealistic family expectations (wanting pain relief with no side effects), an unreasonable fear of addiction, persistent or former drug abuse behavior (rare with end-stage cancer palliation), psychiatric disturbances (depression, anxiety), rapid progression of pain at home with poor caregiver support (caregivers who are not able to appropriately titrate the analgesic dose), or side effects that are not easily controlled.

Successful treatment directed at the tumor may improve pain; a finding of multiple studies is that about three-quarters of patients with cancer pain have some relief when active therapy is

TABLE 8-2	*Common Obstacles to Adequate Analgesia for Cancer Patients*
Side effects of cancer therapy	Chemotherapy and radiation therapy may cause nausea and vomiting, or affect the ability to swallow pills.
Cumulative side effects of therapy	Both opioids and chemotherapy may cause nausea, and vinca alkaloids worsen opioid-induced constipation.
Metabolic abnormalities aggravate medicine side effects	Hypercalcemia, liver dysfunction, or azotemia may enhance constipation, nausea, vomiting, dehydration, and mental changes, narrowing the therapeutic window of opioids.
Tumor effects	Brain metastases affect mobility and cognition making analgesia more difficult. Neutropenia, thrombocytopenia, or infection may interfere with procedures that focus on pain relief.

directed at the tumor (oncologists speak of "palliative chemotherapy"). Some anti-neoplastic drugs are neurotoxic, and may relieve pain by influencing the tumor-host environment even when there is little tumor regression.

Bone metastasis—The most common cause of cancer pain is bone metastasis. This comes as no surprise, as the cancers most likely to metastasize to bone happen to include the most common cancers (breast, prostate, lung, thyroid, and kidney). Radiation therapy may relieve pain without an apparent reduction in tumor size. Bone pain is not completely understood, but suppressing chemical mediators may play a role, as there can be relief before recalcification and bone healing occur. Some patients may wait as long as 8 weeks following treatment to have pain relief. The sensitivity of a particular tumor to local radiotherapy may vary and therefore pain relief may also vary considerably.

Bone pain may be an oncologic emergency. New back pain may indicate a risk of pathological fracture and spinal cord compression and paralysis. This requires immediate attention, usually radiation therapy.

Analgesic therapy—As cancer pain worsens, the initial steps are reasonably straightforward: escalating doses of opioids, use of analgesic adjuvants, manipulating combinations of agents, changing routes of delivery, schedules, and devices (Chapter 2). The use of oral sustained-release tablets or skin reservoir delivery systems may be effective, convenient, and well-tolerated, even in patients with far advanced illness. Experience has demonstrated that patients have a wide range of opioid requirements—we have treated patients with cancer who required as much as 30 grams of morphine per day. Despite patients receiving such high opioid doses, there has been a low incidence of adverse side effects and no increase in mortality.

Effective management of pain starts with an assessment and understanding of the patient's complaint and pain syndrome. The etiology of the pain problem must be accurately defined. Most cancer pain is caused by the cancer itself. Pain can be a side effect of therapy (about one-fifth of "cancer pain"), and a small number of patients have pain unrelated to the cancer (i.e., diabetic neuropathy, herpes zoster, or arthritis). It is important to distinguish between visceral, somatic, and neuropathic pain because management will be different (Chapter 2).

The Last Phase of Illness

The last weeks of life bring dramatic physical and functional changes with increased dependency, frailty, asthenia, and at the end, mental clouding. An analysis of the final days of 275 consecutive patients found that asthenia (90%), anorexia (85%), pain (76%), nausea (68%), and constipation were the most common symptoms (3). Another study of the last 4 weeks of life observed that less than 5% of patients suffered from hallucinations, diarrhea, nightmares, hiccoughs, pruritus, or panic attacks (16). Gender and age had little effect on the prevalence of symptoms during the last days of life. Previously controlled symptoms that escalate often foreshadow the patient's death.

A study of the final hours of 200 consecutive patients found that 91% died "peacefully," and without a crisis such as bleeding, hemoptysis, dyspnea, restlessness, pain, or vomiting (17). Noisy breathing ("death rattle") was common (56%), but easily controlled with anticholinergic drugs. Almost one-third of patients were awake until the time of death, with only 1% unresponsive for more than 48 hours prior to their death.

The painful signs of dying may lead the patient or family to request or demand hospitalization. There is a widespread assumption that dying at home is always better and easier than the hospital, but that is not true for all patients. Those who have been treated in hospice are usually comfortable with death at home. Without hospice support, many families do not understand or are ill-prepared for the burden of nursing the terminally ill patient. Left at home, they may feel abandoned by the health care system.

When death is imminent, there should be less concern for potential adverse effects of symptom control therapy (i.e., the gastric effects of steroids or non-steroidal anti-inflammatory drugs, opioids masking abdominal pain, acetaminophen masking fever). It may be appropriate to eliminate as much medication for non-problematic concomitant disease (i.e., hypertension or diabetes). Doctors are occasionally concerned about analgesics hampering the patient's ability to communicate with the family. In such cases, you may let the family and patient guide you (they usually want adequate pain control).

When death is imminent, the moral distinction between allowing the patient to die and possibly hastening death (short of frank euthanasia) appears less meaningful. For example, there is little to be gained by forcing nutrition and hydration in the face of cachexia, even though withholding them may hasten death. There is rarely sustained reversal of symptoms with hydration, and the extra fluid can add to discomfort (aggravating edema or congestion, or increasing urination so that a catheter is needed). Let the patient be your guide. If there is no request for food or water do not force it; tube feeding and/or intravenous hydration are inappropriate. In the last days and hours of life thirst is an infrequent symptom, and it is common for patients to drink little. At this stage of management, all decisions should be based on the patient's comfort, and not on longevity.

References

1. Jemal A, Thomas A. Cancer Statistics 2002;52:1.
2. Slevins ML. Making decisions about palliative chemotherapy. ASCO Education Book, 1992. 28th meeting:118.
3. Bruera E, Sweeny C, Calder K, et al. Patient preferences vs. physician perceptions of therapeutic decisions in cancer care. J Clin Oncol 2001;19:2883–2885.
4. Christakis N, Lamont E. Extent and determinants of error in doctors' prognoses in terminally ill patients: prospective cohort study. BMJ 2000;320:469–472.
5. Llobera J, Esteva M. Terminal cancer: duration and prediction of survival time. Eur J Can 2000;36:2036–2043.

6. Seidman AD, Portenoy R. Quality of life in phase II trials. J Nat Cancer Inst 1991;87:1316.

7. Brescia FJ, Portenoy RK, Ryan M, et al. Pain, opioid use and survival in hospitalized patients with advanced cancer. J Clin Oncol 1992;10: 149–155.

8. Kodish E, Post SG. Oncology and hope. J Clin Oncol 1995;13:1817–1822.

9. Delvecchio MJ, Good BJ, Schaffer C, Lind SE. American oncology and the discourse on hope. Cult Med Psychiatry 1990;14:59–79.

10. Non-small cell lung cancer expert panel (ASCO). Clinical practice guidelines for the treatment of unresectable non-small cell lung cancer. J Clin Oncol 1997;15:2996–3018.

11. Daugherty C, Ratain MJ, Growchowski E. Perceptions of cancer patients and their physicians involved in Phase I trials. J Clin Oncol 1995;13:1062–1072.

12. Cleeland CS, Gonin R, Hatfield AK, et al. Pain and its treatment in outpatients with metastatic cancer. N Engl J Med 1994;330:592–596.

13. Zhukovsky DS. Unmet analgesic needs in cancer patients. J Pain Symptom Manage 1995;10:113–119.

14. Von Roenn JH, Cleeland CS, Gonin R, et al. Physicians' attitudes and practice in cancer pain management. Ann Int Med 1993;119:121–126.

15. Cherny NI, Coyle N, Foley KM. Guidelines in the care of the dying cancer patient. Heme Oncol Clin North Am 1996;10:261–288.

16. Coyle N, Adelhardt J. Character of terminal illness in the advanced cancer patient: pain and other symptoms during the last four weeks of life. J Pain Symptoms Manage 1990;5:83.

17. Enck RE. The final moments. In: Enck RE, ed. The medical care of terminally ill patients. Baltimore: Johns Hopkins University Press, 2002.

9 | *Liver Disease*

George J. Taylor

Liver disease is the tenth leading cause of death in the United States, responsible for more than 25,000 deaths each year (1). Alcoholic liver disease and chronic viral hepatitis account for a majority of cases. Regardless of the etiology, most patients end their lives with cirrhosis complicated by some combination of ascites, jaundice, encephalopathy, gastroesophageal varices, or hepatorenal syndrome.

Natural history and prognosis

While most heavy drinkers develop fatty infiltration of the liver, just one-fourth develops cirrhosis. Many of these never become symptomatic; 40% die from another illness before cirrhosis is clinically apparent (data from autopsy studies) (2,3). Following inoculation with hepatitis C virus (HCV), 80% become chronically infected, and 20% develop cirrhosis (4).

After cirrhosis develops, median survival is 6 years. In the Study to Understand Prognoses and Preferences for Outcomes and Risks of Treatment (SUPPORT), estimation of imminent mortality was more reliable for end-stage liver disease than it was for heart failure or chronic lung disease, but somewhat less reliable than it was for lung cancer (5). Clinical and laboratory features that indicate limited short-term survival are also, in general, the indications for liver transplantation (Table 9-1). While transplantation successfully alters the natural history—is life saving—less than one-fourth of those with advanced disease has it done. Contraindications prevent many from having transplant, and a limited number of organs play a role as well. Thus, most patients with end-stage liver disease die from the illness, and at some point benefit from palliative care.

Most of the therapies for complications of liver disease may also be considered palliative. When might the patient be considered terminal, or at a stage of illness when hospice care is warranted? Patients with cirrhosis and ascites who become severely jaundiced or who have progressively rising bilirubin have poor short-term survival. That is also the case for those with

TABLE 9-1	*Liver Transplantation**

Indications for Liver Transplantation
(A combination of these features identifies the patient with end-stage disease.)

Biochemical
    Serum bilirubin >5 mg/dL**
    Prothrombin time elevated
    Serum albumin <2.5 g/dL
Clinical and quality of life
    Severe or progressive hepatic encephalopathy
    Refractory ascites
    Recurrent spontaneous bacterial peritonitis
    Recurrent portal hypertensive bleed (varices)
    Progressive fatigue or malnutrition (usually with ascites)
    Hepatorenal syndrome
    Recurrent biliary sepsis
    Intractable pruritus

Absolute Contraindications to Liver Transplantation
HIV seropositivity (often progresses to full-blown AIDS after transplant; the effect
    of antiviral therapy is uncertain at present)
Extrahepatic malignancy and some hepatobiliary cancers
Uncontrolled sepsis
Active alcoholism or substance abuse (must be sober >6 months)
Irreversible neurological disease (see discussion of encephalopathy)
Advanced heart or lung disease
Inability to comply with immunosuppression protocol
Anatomic abnormalities

Relative Contraindications
Advanced age
Portal vein thrombosis
Previous extrahepatic malignancy
Prior portosystemic shunting (can make surgery difficult; TIPS does not, see text)
Renal failure (note that hepatorenal syndrome usually improves)
Severe obesity
Malnutrition

---

* The indications for transplantation are clinical features that also identify the patient with
a poor near-term prognosis. Those who need transplantation but cannot have it because of
contraindications may thus be assumed to have end-stage liver disease (1).
** With cholestatic liver disease (i.e., primary biliary cirrhosis or sclerosing cholangitis) the
threshold bilirubin is higher. These patients have more pruritus, metabolic bone disease,
and biliary sepsis.

hepatic encephalopathy or hepatorenal syndrome who are resistant to conventional therapy.

Communicating with the patient and family

The general principles of communicating with the patient and family outlined in Chapter 1 are worth reviewing and apply to the patient with chronic liver disease. When it is clear that short-term survival is limited, do not put off the discussion of treatment options with the patient and family. Encephalopathy can develop, making it impossible for the patient to make decisions. Other complications of liver disease, such as hepatorenal syndrome and spontaneous bacterial peritonitis, may also affect mental status.

The doctor must first educate the patient and family about the nature of the illness. As an opener, many find it useful to ask the patient what he understands about the condition. In addition to letting you know where to start, it sets the stage for dialogue rather than monologue. In the course of the discussion you should learn important things about the patient and his family (i.e., who can be expected to provide support, or where there is a need for reconciliation), and about the patient's goals and expectations.

There is information you must transmit about what to expect with end-stage liver disease. Consider the sample conversation in Box 9-1. This format is a bit artificial, as it is a monologue with no input from the patient or family. But it does cover issues that are related to management decisions and advance directives. In ideal circumstances, decisions develop through a series of conversations, and these conversations include more than just the medical issues.

Palliation: syndromes and symptoms

Pain—The chronic phase of cirrhosis is not usually painful. Opioids and sedatives may precipitate hepatic encephalopathy and should be avoided or used with caution when they are needed for coexisting conditions. Nonsteroidal anti-inflammatory drugs, including aspirin, may trigger renal insufficiency. Acetaminophen is a good choice for minor discomfort. It is hepatotoxic at high doses, but less than 3 gm/day is safe for patients with cirrhosis (6).

In contrast, pain is a common feature of terminal cirrhosis and ascites. Patients become uncomfortable with abdominal bloating, cramps, and pain. In the SUPPORT study, the degree of pain among those with liver disease was comparable to that

BOX 9-1	*A conversation with a patient with advanced liver disease*

"Your liver condition has reached a stage where we call it 'cirrhosis of the liver.' This usually means that the liver has scarring, and the scar tissue blocks blood flow. Blood backs up behind the liver, and the pressure of this causes fluid to build up in the abdomen. The fluid is called 'ascites.'

"We have good treatments for ascites, and believe we can control it. At some point, we may reach a time where other complications of the liver disease develop that we cannot control. These complications can be fatal. That time is not just around the corner, but it is important we discuss what may happen so that you and your family can plan your care. It would be important, for example, to avoid treatments that have no chance of working and at the same time make you uncomfortable.

"There are a couple of situations I have in mind: First, some— not all but some—people develop changes in brain function, called encephalopathy. We have good medicine to control this, but it can reach a stage where the medicine does not work, and there is coma. At that point in your life, you will have little pain or suffering—and what there is can be controlled. You would die peacefully. A second condition is kidney failure caused by the liver condition—again, a problem that some, but not all, people with liver disease get. This also can be fatal and eventually is not treatable. It does not respond to dialysis (the kidney machine). Like encephalopathy, it is not painful, and usually leads to a peaceful death. In both cases, keeping you alive artificially, with breathing machines, tube feedings, IVs, and treatment of infections cannot help you survive the illness.

"In such cases—when nothing can be done to prolong life— most people decide to avoid hopeless treatments that prolong what suffering there is, and instead to choose treatments that control symptoms like pain. The good news is that we have good medicines to control most symptoms, and I do not believe that you will have that much pain. It is for sure that I will stick with you to do the best I can to help you through this.

"You and your family need to make some decisions, and work on advance directives. You will want to think of the limits you want to set so that you avoid uncomfortable procedures at this stage of your life. I am here to give you my best advice, but these are decisions you will make. I will support whatever you decide."

experienced with lung or colon cancer, and considerably worse than discomfort experienced with heart or lung disease (5).

Undertreatment of pain with advanced liver disease is common for a variety of reasons. Many of these patients are alcoholics, and physicians are reluctant to prescribe narcotics when there is a history of substance abuse. Hepatic failure may affect drug metabolism, again influencing doctors to undertreat. Compared with other diseases, doctors have been reluctant to identify patients with liver disease as terminally ill, and thus are slower to shift into a palliative model of care. In medical school we are taught to avoid opiods for abdominal pain of uncertain cause so that we do not mask the evolving surgical abdomen, and the etiology of pain with end-stage liver disease is often uncertain. Finally, these patients tend to be younger than those dying from other chronic illnesses, another barrier to the recognition of the illness as end-stage. We are reluctant to have a young patient become opioid dependent.

Patients and families sense all of this, and have concern about pain control. None of the above is a good excuse for avoiding adequate pain relief. In the terminal patient, it is unlikely that you will be masking the acute, surgical abdomen. While spontaneous peritonitis is a common complication, it tends to be asymptomatic.

The principles of pain management are those outlined in Chapter 2. Carefully titrating the dose and dosing interval allows the safe use of opioids. Alcoholic patients often crave alcohol at the final stages of cirrhosis, and there is no reason to exclude modest alcohol consumption from the comfort care regimen (a couple ounces of spirits per day).

Ascites—This is the leading cause of decompensation, and develops in about one-third of patients who have had cirrhosis for 10 years (2). Ambulatory patients with a first episode of ascites have a 3-year mortality of 50%, and when ascites become refractory, half die within a year (7).

Ascites can develop in patients with diseased peritoneum or abdominal organs (i.e., abdominal malignancy, pancreatitis, or tuberculosis in a setting of AIDS). In such cases the ascitic fluid is an exudate, with an elevated protein (8). Like the edema and effusions of congestive heart failure, the mechanism of ascites with portal hypertension is increased hydrostatic pressure. There is little protein in the fluid—it is transudative. Thus, a simple test that helps determine the pathophysiology of ascites is measurement albumin in serum and the ascitic fluid. With cirrhosis and other forms of portal hypertension (including Budd-Chiari syndrome, cardiac cirrhosis, and portal vein thrombosis) the serum albumen is much higher than the ascitic fluid albumin. A serum-ascites albumen ratio above 1.1 suggests portal hypertension, the usual case with end-stage liver disease with cirrhosis and ascites.

Treatment options are outlined in Table 9-2, beginning with the least aggressive approach. Subsequent steps are added; salt restriction and diuretics are helpful even when more aggressive measures are being used. Sodium restriction is most effective for those with elevated urinary sodium excretion. Peripheral edema is an important finding; when present aggressive diuresis is possible as there is rapid exchange of fluid between edema and the vascular space. When absent, the patient cannot mobilize more than 1 L of fluid per day—movement of fluid between ascites and the vascular space is "slow." Pushing harder with diuretics results in contraction of vascular volume and renal insufficiency.

When renal function is normal, spironolactone is more effective than loop diuretics; start with 50–100 mg/day and push the dose to 400 mg/day. It is metabolized by the liver, and a steady state may not be reached for 2 weeks. Once daily dosing is adequate.

Failing to respond to spironolactone or the presence of azotemia indicate a need to add a loop diuretic. Furosemide is our first choice, but when there is resistance to therapy we shift

TABLE 9-2	*Treatment of Ascites*

Step 1 Sodium restriction (effective if urinary sodium is high); abstinence from alcohol

Step 2 Add diuretics; first spironolactone, then a loop diuretic (see text). Goal = 1 L diuresis (1 kg weight loss) per day if there is no edema, or more rapid weight loss if there is peripheral edema. Fluid restriction if there is hyponatremia. Possibly bed rest.*

Step 3 Add large volume paracentesis (LVP, see text), and continue diuretic therapy.

Step 4 Portal decompression (TIPS), or peritoneovenous shunt for selected patients.

Step 5 Indwelling drain for palliation if life expectancy is less than 3 weeks.

* Bed rest facilitates diuresis but creates other problems; on balance we prefer continued activity and going to Steps 3–4 for ascites control in order to maintain conditioning.

quickly to a newer generation agent, bumetanide or torsemide. The newer loop diuretics are more easily and predictably absorbed, and thus are more reliable when there is splanchnic edema (note the discussion of diuretic therapy in Chapter 3).

Just 10% of patients with ascites develop resistance to diuretics and salt restriction, but refractory ascites is a common feature of end-stage disease. Large volume paracentesis (LVP) is the next step in treatment, usually serial 5 L taps at 1- to 2-day intervals. To avoid hypotension, stop diuretics for a week before LVP. If that is not possible, or for the patient with azotemia, consider colloid support (usually albumin, 5–8 grams intravenously for each liter of ascites removed).

An indwelling catheter to drain re-accumulating ascitic fluid may be considered at the end of life, when estimated survival is less than 3 weeks. Longer use leads to excessive malnutrition and reduced vascular volume.

Surgical methods for draining ascites (peritoneovenous shunts), or reducing portal hypertension (portocaval shunting), may be effective as the next step to control ascites, and may be considered for palliation. The preferred technique is transjugular intrahepatic protosystemic shunt (TIPS), as it is nonsurgical. Comparison trials have not shown a survival benefit of TIPS over LVP, so it is used when LVP is no longer effective or not possible (i.e., a patient with abdominal adhesions who cannot be tapped, or one without access to a facility that can do it). TIPS can precipitate hepatic encephalopathy; a rare patient must have the shunt reversed. TIPS is contraindicated when there is pulmonary hypertension or right heart failure, and in patients with sepsis, hepatic neoplasm, or portal vein thrombosis. With severe, end-stage hepatic failure (e.g., tense ascites and rising bilirubin), TIPS has little to offer.

Hepatic encephalopathy—The earliest symptoms are changes in mood or disorderd sleep (9). This progresses to confusion or lethargy, and eventually, to coma. Physical findings include shifting neurologic signs such as asterixis, hyperreflexia, or rigidity. Asterixis is usually present, but is nonspecific and may occur with other metabolic disorders.

Though serum ammonia often is elevated, this is a clinical diagnosis which requires the presence of liver disease and the exclusion of other disorders (Table 9-3). Early in the course of liver disease, encephalopathy may be easily controlled with medical therapy (Table 9-3) (9). However, as a feature of end-stage liver

TABLE 9-3	*Treatment of Hepatic Encephalopathy*
Exclude other causes of altered mental status	Acute intoxication, sedative overdose, delirium tremens, Wernicke's encephalopathy, subdural hematoma, meningitis, hypoglycemia, etc.
Treat precipitating factors	GI bleeding, sepsis (possibly SBP), electrolyte disturbance (from diuretics or excess catharsis), dehydration, excessive protein intake, CNS active drugs, constipation. If post-shunt is unresponsive to medical therapy, may have to reverse the shunt.
Protein restriction	Less than 60 g/day.
Lactulose orally or as an enema to induce catharsis	Give enough to induce diarrhea initially, then give it 1–4 times daily to produce 4 stools/day. This works as an osmotic laxative, and it lowers stool pH (converting ammonia to the poorly absorbed ammonium ion). Some do not tolerate the bloating. With a first episode of encephalopathy, 90% improve in two days.
If no improvement, add antibiotics (start with neomycin)	Reduces intestinal ammonia production by bacteria. Watch for renal toxicity with neomycin, which is not completely "nonabsorbable." Similar results are possible with chronic tetracycline or metronidazole therapy.

SBP = spontaneous bacterial peritonitis.

failure or when it is chronic and irreversible, encephalopathy progresses to coma and is a terminal condition.

An important decision for the patient or surrogate decision-maker is treatment when encephalopathy fails to respond to usual measures. When the patient is no longer able to eat or drink, tube feeding or parenteral nutrition offer little chance for meaningful recovery. This should be considered when writing advance directives, and many patients elect to decline tube feeding and intravenous hydration in the event of unresponsive encephalopathy or hepatic coma (Box 9-1).

Spontaneous bacterial peritonitis—Patients with ascites are susceptible to spontaneous bacterial peritonitis (SBP); low albumen level in ascitic fluid increases the risk of infection (8). Migration of bacteria through the bowel wall and into lymphatics and veins is the apparent route of infection. Some patients develop fever and abdominal pain, but an absence of symptoms is just as common. The diagnosis may be suspected with increasing jaundice or encephalopathy. Paracentesis is needed to make the diagnosis. Spontaneous bacterial peritonitis may be a terminal complication, and may be considered when discussing advance directives with the patient and family. At some stage of advanced liver disease, and depending on other symptoms, a patient or his surrogate might decide to avoid antibiotic therapy. For example, this may be a rational decision for a person with persistent encephalopathy and refractory ascites (Box 9-1).

Jaundice and pruritus—Elevated bilirubin is a feature of advanced liver disease, regardless of the etiology. It is a prominent feature of cirrhosis caused by hepatitis C, and is most severe with cholestatic liver diseases (primary biliary cirrhosis and sclerosing cholangitis).

A rise in bilirubin, even with chronic liver disease, should prompt a search for mechanical obstruction (e.g., gallstone or extrinsic constriction of the bile ducts). With obstruction excluded, a progressive increase in bilirubin usually indicates poor short-term prognosis.

The worst side effect of high bilirubin is pruritus (1). It may be severe enough to warrant transplantation. The pathogenesis is uncertain, but a response to cholestyramine implicates bile salts. Either cholestyramine or colestipol can be used, and the advantage of the latter is twice daily rather than four times daily dosing. Fortunately, 90% of patients respond to bile acid binding.

There are a large number of therapies that have been tried for the remaining 10% (1). Antihistamines can be pushed to the point of sedation, and are useful at night for this reason. Rifampicin has been effective in a randomized trial, and ursodeoxycholic acid has helped those with primary biliary cirrhosis. An effect of opioid antagonists indicates a central mechanism of pruritus; naloxone works but is a parenteral drug. Two oral agents, nalmefene and naltrexone, have been effective in clinical trials.

Hepatorenal syndrome—Before making this diagnosis other causes of renal dysfunction should be excluded, including obstructive uropathy, volume depletion, acute tubular necrosis, glomerulonephritis, and drug-induced nephropathy (10). With hepatorenal syndrome the kidneys are normal, and the mechanism of azotemia is vasoconstriction and hypoperfusion. Patients with portal hypertension have decreased intravascular volume, and renal perfusion is dependent on prostaglandin-mediated vasodilatation. Non-steroidal inflammatory drugs are prostaglandin-blockers, and thus should be avoided by patients with advanced liver disease.

Hepatorenal syndrome is more likely to occur when there is aggressive diuresis, large volume paracentesis, hyponatremia, low blood pressure, and spontaneous peritonitis. Supporting the diagnosis is low urine sodium and a normal urinary sediment.

Volume expansion is the treatment when urine volume falls and creatinine rises. Beyond that there is no effective therapy. An occasional patient responds to TIPS (an area of ongoing research). Dialysis has not been found to improve survival. Like hepatic encephalopathy, when simple measures fail, hepatorenal syndrome may prove to be the terminal illness.

Varices and variceal bleeding—Esophageal varices are collateral channels between the portal and systemic venous circulations (11). About one-third of them bleed, usually those near the gastroesophageal junction. Bleeding is most common when they are large (Laplace law at work), and when portal pressure is especially high. Alcoholic patients who continue drinking, and who have poor liver function are more likely to bleed.

Therapy to reduce portal pressure can prevent bleeding from varices. Beta blockade lowers splanchic flow and portal pressure, and may reduce the incidence of bleeding 40% to 50%. Adding isosorbide mononitrate provides further benefit. While effective, many with advanced cirrhosis cannot tolerate the beta blockers, much less the beta blocker-nitrate combination.

Endoscopic procedures have proved useful in eradicating varices. Sclerotherapy has been replaced by band ligation. This is more effective than beta blockade as prophylaxis against bleeding. Emergence of this approach is an argument for endoscopic screening of patients with severe cirrhosis.

When bleeding occurs, it can be massive but usually is painless. First line therapy is pharmacologic (11). Somatostatin, or its synthetic analogue, octreotide, stops bleeding in 80% of cases. These drugs have few side effects and require no special monitoring; the mechanism of action is uncertain (11). Vasopressin reduces splanchnic flow; while effective, it may cause generalized vasospasm, including mesenteric or myocardial ischemia. Endoscopic treatment effectively controls bleeding in 90%, and the results with sclerotherapy and banding are similar. Balloon tamponade is rarely needed, and is now used as a rescue device to stabilize the patient. When all else fails, lowering portal pressure with TIPS can prevent recurrent bleeding.

Thus, we now have effective treatment for esophageal varices and bleeding. Nevertheless, short-term prognosis is terrible when bleeding occurs late in the course of liver disease, at a time when there is multiorgan failure (e.g., liver disease plus renal disease or encephalopathy). At this stage of the illness, TIPS may prevent recurrent bleeding, but no one survives a month (11). Terminal variceal bleeding is at least painless, and any discomfort is easily controlled with opioids. The biggest problem is that it is so distressful for the family.

References

1. Saab S, Han S, Martin P. Liver transplantation; selection, listing criteria and preoperative management. Clin Liver Dis 2000;4:513–532.
2. D'Amico G, Morabito A, Pagliaro L, et al. Survival and prognostic indicators in compensated and decompensated cirrhosis. Dig Dis Sci 1986;31:468–475.
3. Gines P, Quintero E, Arroyo V, et al. Compensated cirrhosis: natural history and prognostic factors. Hepatology 1987;7:122–128.
4. Cheney CP. Hepatitis C. Infect Dis Clin North Am 2000;14:633–667.
5. Roth K, Lynn J, Zhong Z, et al. Dying with end stage liver disease with cirrhosis: insights from SUPPORT. J Am Geriats Soc 2000;48:S122–S130.
6. Sandowski S, Runyon B. Hepatobiliary disease: cirrhosis. Clin In Fam Pract 2000;2:59–77.
7. Salerno F, Gianmario B, Moser P, et al. Survival and prognostic factors of cirrhotic patients with ascites. Am J Gastro 1993;88:514–519.
8. Reynolds T. Ascites. Clin Liver Dis 2000;4151–4168.
9. Riordan S, Williams R. Treatment of hepatic encephalopathy. N Engl J Med 1997;337:473–479.
10. Bataller R, Gines P, Arroyo V, Rodes J. Hepatorenal syndrome. Clin Liver Dis 2000;4:487–502.
11. Sharara A, Rocker D. Gastroesophageal variceal hemorrhage. N Engl J Med 2001;345:669–681.

10 | *The Pediatric Patient*

Dale Ann Singer

Death after infancy is more likely to be the result of an accident or a violent event than due to a medical illness (Figure 10-1a and b) (1). Because of medical progress, family medicine specialists and pediatricians can practice for months or years without caring for a dying child. Our experience with death before adulthood is more often through television, movies, the arts, and literature than in daily experience. Young people who die seem to be someone else's children, someone else's patients.

When treating end-stage heart, kidney, or lung disease or malignancy, the medical issues are similar for children and adults. Principles of palliation also are the same, though medication doses must be adjusted for the patient's size. This chapter will not review the medical conditions that have been the subject of previous chapters, but instead will discuss other issues that are unique to children: Parents and guardians must make choices for patients who will die before acquiring the maturity and skills needed to participate fully in the decision-making process. Young patients continue to grow and mature during their final weeks and months of life. Children often continue their education and participate in extracurricular activities both in school and in the community despite having severe life-limiting illness. These young patients may need special services to allow meaningful inclusion in the activities of childhood. Teachers, coaches, and activities directors may be frightened to have these children in the classroom, in youth groups and activities, or on playing fields.

Many physicians, including pediatricians, feel they have inadequate formal training in end-of-life care, although that is changing. Pediatric hospice services are increasingly available.

The patient population is diverse

The child may be a previously healthy 11-day-old, 11-month-old, 11-year-old, or 16-year-old child who sustains head trauma, is comatose, and requires ventilator support. Or, the patient may be a 13-month-old toddler on renal dialysis who would benefit from kidney transplant or a 13-year-old patient with renal failure since

Leading Causes of Death in Children (Ages 1 to 14) in the United States, 1997

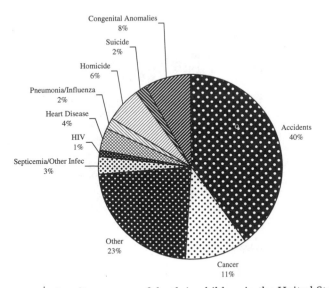

FIGURE 10-1a | Leading causes of death in children in the United States, 1997. Causes of death among children 1 to 14 years (death data are from the National Center for Health Statistics public-use file).

early childhood who refuses further dialysis or a third kidney transplant. Perhaps the child is a relatively medically sophisticated 6-, 11-, or 15-year-old with leukemia recurrent soon after bone marrow transplant who wants to volunteer for experimental therapy. The patient may be a 3-month-old, 3-year-old, or 13-year-old graduate of a newborn intensive care unit with irreversible chronic lung disease, short gut syndrome, significant developmental delay, seizure disorder, and cerebral palsy. These patients can benefit from extending comprehensive pediatric care to the end of life.

The physician's role

Pediatricians are trained to care for the maturing patient within the context of his or her family and community. They know their patients, families, and the resources available. It is their professional obligation, therefore, to coordinate the care of their patients who will die before reaching adulthood. The physicians

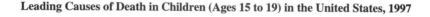

Leading Causes of Death in Children (Ages 15 to 19) in the United States, 1997

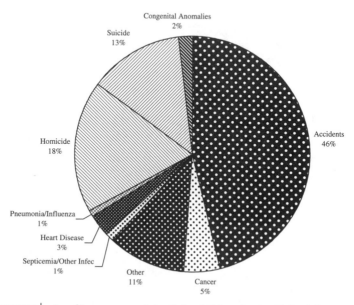

Congenital Anomalies
2%

Suicide
13%

Homicide
18%

Pneumonia/Influenza
1%

Heart Disease
3%

Septicemia/Other Infec
1%

Other
11%

Cancer
5%

Accidents
46%

FIGURE 10-1b | Leading causes of death in children in the United States, 1997. Causes of death among adolescents 15 to 19 years (death data are from the National Center for Health Statistics public-use file).

involved may be pediatric sub-specialists caring for a child and/or general pediatricians.

As the child's doctor, you will work with parents; guardians; nurses; counselors; social workers; child life specialists; physical, occupational, and speech therapists; educators; volunteers; and others. Central to comprehensive pediatric care is respect for each young person as a unique individual with family and community associations. You should identify the child's goals for the future, however limited the goals or the expected future may be. You also need to know the family and its aspirations for the child. As part of this, you must respect the moral and religious beliefs of the patient, family, and community.

It is important to sense and acknowledge conflict in the family. The health care team should help the family resolve this before the young patient dies. The time and effort required may be considerable. However, active conflict contributes to the suffering of the dying child or adolescent. If unsettled, it is a burden to survivors.

The physician is responsible for informing the patient and the family of the medical situation and the expected course of the illness with accuracy and sensitivity. You must help decide when the goal of care should shift from cure to palliation. Palliative care must then be effective, with adequate pain and symptom control. An important role of the pediatrician is management of anxiety and depression (as experienced by the patient, family, and others on the health care team). Reassessment needs to be ongoing as the patient's medical condition changes and the options for intervention shift. The attending pediatrician is responsible for updating patients and families regarding the response to treatment and the implications for morbidity and mortality (2).

While providing care for the child, you have an important responsibility to educate parents, siblings, extended family members, and health care and educational personnel. All of them should understand the illness and the treatment plan, and this is especially important as the disease approaches its terminal stage. Often the child is overlooked, but, as the patient, needs education as well. Those with chronic and eventually fatal conditions need to learn about the illness starting at an early age.

Young patients should be taught to participate in their own medical care and decision-making. Ideally this process starts during routine pediatric care, long before a child approaches the end of life. Physicians can teach parents how to include their children in medical decisions without abdicating either their responsibility or authority.

Communicating with the patient and family and making decisions

Physicians recommend care to patients or their designated decision-makers who may accept, modify, or reject these recommendations. Usually, recommendations are made after considerable education and discussion with a patient and family. Nurses, counselors, social workers, other members of the medical team, extended family members, clergy, or close friends may help clarify the issues and offer support. Medical team members and family support people who may help with decision-making should be invited to participate in the discussions if the patient and family agree.

The general principles of communication reviewed throughout this text apply in the pediatric setting (note the discussion in

Chapter 1). The first goal is to help the patient and family understand the illness, accepting that the level of understanding will vary with the level of medical sophistication. Your vocabulary should be appropriate; this is not the time to use the passive voice or to speak of "treatment modalities" (Is there ever a time for such jargon?). With children you may find it helpful to start with a description of the organ system that is involved (i.e., "The kidneys get rid of extra water and other liquids you drink, so that you do not swell up. They also get rid of other things your body makes that are not good for you if they build up—like 'urea,' which your body makes when you eat and then digest foods with protein, like meat, beans, or bread.").

Even medically unsophisticated people are capable of comprehending the major issues, including treatment alternatives and prognosis. As has been emphasized throughout this text, processing complicated new information may require multiple discussions. Do not assume that you have communicated adequately when you have discussed it only one time.

While it is important to be sensitive to the feelings of parents who are suffering with their child, it is important to honestly define the prognosis. Giving false hope can be crueler than providing the truth, and it is unethical. At some point a "family meeting" may be helpful. It is an efficient way to relay information to parents and other interested parties, it carries the weight of an "official forum," and by its nature, it conveys the doctor's commitment to good communication. Although others may be involved, it should be clear that the patient and parents or guardians will be making the ultimate decisions.

The patient must be the central figure in the decision process, but the child-patient commonly defers to the parent. This may be the case in the final hours or days of life, at a time when further medical intervention is futile. Continuing with additional diagnostic testing or treatment may extend life for an interval, but cannot restore health. Children and adolescents often wait for permission to "stop fighting" from their parents or other family members.

For a patient who has suffered brain death but continues with a heart beat and adequate tissue perfusion with mechanical ventilation, timing of cessation of support is left to the attending physician. If the patient's tissues and organs are to be donated for transplantation, there is usually a protocol for tissue collection and then discontinuing support. Otherwise, an attending physician must decide when and how to disconnect the ventilator, IV medication, and monitors with sensitivity to the family's needs.

When the outcome is inevitable, but the life span is uncertain—
Some children have lethal conditions recognized early in life. They benefit from routine pediatric care, as well as subspecialty consultation for complicated medical problems. Take, for example, a newborn intensive care unit graduate with irreversible bronchopulmonary dysplasia, short gut syndrome, severe developmental delay, seizure disorder, and cerebral palsy. The parents may decide that supportive care is appropriate. However, they may also decide that, in the event of a cardiac or pulmonary arrest, resuscitation is not in the best interest of their child. Year after year, the child lives despite the poor prognosis. The doctor and family must decide whether or not to provide routine childhood immunizations, treat potentially life threatening bacterial infectious illnesses with antibiotics, proceed with elective surgeries, or other interventions.

Pediatricians and parents are faced with the reality that not every child can be cared for in the home throughout their entire lives. Sometimes it is in the best interest of the child to be cared for in a medical foster home or institution. The patient may eventually outlive his parents or their resources, physically and emotionally. The pediatrician is responsible for reassessment of the patient and for recommendations that reflect the current situation. With the doctor's support, the parents must choose care that is most appropriate for their child.

Competent pediatric patients and those acquiring competence—
There are generally accepted criteria for competence to make medical decisions in young patients. These include an established values system, an ability to understand treatment options including their benefits and risks, and an understanding of the consequences of choices (3). It is generally agreed that an adolescent of 14 years of age has acquired moral development with identifiable, consistent values and is able to participate fully in the medical decision-making process. Adolescents may seek the advice of parents or others, but a competent 14-year-old patient must accept or reject the elements of a treatment care plan (4).

An adolescent patient who is unable to make decisions is no different from an adult in the same circumstances, and is dependent upon surrogate decision-makers. This is often the case with acute neurologic injury or chronic disease.

Few adolescents 14 and older have written advance directives that provide instructions in the event of fluctuating competence or permanent loss of decision-making capacity. However, if the patient made his wishes known prior to his accident in discussions with parents, family, friends, teachers, or clergy, the doctor and surrogate decision-makers have a moral and legal obligation to honor these choices as if the young patient were an adult. The patient may have indicated that his choice would be to continue therapy, despite very minimal chance for recovery. Or, he may have requested withdrawing ventilator support if the outcome is virtually certain to be permanent coma or persistent vegetative state. He may have felt using his organs for transplantation would be something he wanted to do. Fourteen years is the accepted age for acquisition of competence to make these medical decisions. Eighteen years of age is an arbitrary legal definition of adulthood in many states (5).

Most often, an adolescent has not seriously considered the issues or reached enduring decisions. If the neurologically impaired patient is expected to recover decision-making capacity and his wishes are unknown, many physicians feel an obligation to continue to provide supportive care for a period of time until the outcome is more certain. Once the clinical course has better defined the outcome, a decision must be made for the patient if recovery of decision-making capacity is no longer deemed likely. A surrogate decision-maker acts in the best interest of the patient. Usually the parents are recognized as guardians and assume this responsibility. When there is consensus among parents and significant friends as to what the patient would have wanted, physicians should base recommendations for further care on choices that are most likely to have been consistent with the patient's wishes.

There can be conflict within the family about life-sustaining therapy. Take, for example, a 13-year-old boy with renal failure since early childhood who refuses further dialysis or a third renal transplant. Given the duration of his illness, he is capable of understanding his situation. His dissent must be taken seriously, and, if supported by his parents, his choice must be respected. In most cases like this, parents comply with the wishes of their child. But what if one parent agrees with him, but the other insists on continued aggressive care? It may be easier when the child has reached the age of medical competence (14 years old), but even then minors require the permission of their guardians, and such conflicts may be difficult to resolve. As a mediator, the doctor can only present the medical options, with the prognosis for each alternative, listening to the viewpoints of the parties involved in the decision, and making a recommendation for a treatment plan that is in the best interests of the child. Nurses, social workers, counselors, and psychologists are often helpful, and your hospital's Medical Ethics Committee can be of assistance in resolving such conflicts.

Even if both parents and the child agree to withhold dialysis, the patient continues to need end-of-life medical care, and the family needs ongoing information and support. A limited period of dialysis may be indicated to allow time to resolve the conflict or for the child to say goodbye to extended family members and friends (note the discussion of short-term dialysis support in Chapter 5). The child and family need to understand what medical interventions are most likely to help the child remain pain free, alert, and interactive for the greatest length of time, if that is their wish. The pediatrician is responsible for putting together a team of physicians, nurses, social workers, and others that will provide the patient and family with appropriate help whether the patient is to die at home, in the hospital, or in a hospice setting.

Clinical trials—Experimental therapies and clinical studies offer special challenges. Consider a 15-year-old girl with recurrent leukemia soon after bone marrow transplant who is likely to die from her disease or complications. She is an experienced patient well aware of the issues (6). Such an individual is considered competent to consent to experimental therapy, with parental permission, or to refuse this or any other life-sustaining interventions.

The pediatrician as the clinical investigator is responsible for identifying patients for clinical trials. The possibility of conflict between this vested interest and the patient's best interest is an ethical issue that must be recognized (i.e., Is the doctor paid a fee or otherwise rewarded for enrolling patients?). Making decisions in such circumstances can be difficult. Using the best information available, the adolescent patient, her family, and the doctor must balance the reality of eventual death from the malignancy against the potential benefits and risks of untested agents. The doctor anticipates gaining knowledge with the research study, but there may be little value for the patient (note the discussion of clinical trials in Chapter 8). For example, some clinical trials are designed to determine toxic levels of new medicines, and not intended as therapy. Of course, supportive care must be the first priority, and patients and their parents should be clearly informed about the goals and expectations of a clinical trial (7).

Many 7- to 14-year-old patients with recurrent leukemia have gained, during the course of a long illness, the maturity and skills necessary to make an informed decision. They can volunteer for an unproven, experimental therapy, within the context of a clinical trial, with parental permission. These young patients usually cling to the hope that the new interventions will offer them cure. If their physician has educated them well, they can retain this hope while understanding that the expectation of an experimental therapy is for palliation, hopefully without significant toxicities. These young, experienced, relatively mature children are often the best judges of when an experimental therapy becomes excessively burdensome. Children, like adults, are often willing to take high risks despite overwhelmingly poor odds. It is ethical to allow them to do so when they have demonstrated consistent values, understanding of the benefits and risks of treatment, and the probable consequences of their decisions.

Patients without the ability to consent or assent—Infants and children less than 7 years of age generally have a limited ability to participate meaningfully in major decisions about health care. Even children 7 through 13 years of age may be unable to participate meaningfully if they lack any prior experience with significant illness or injury. Their parents or guardians give permission for care based on their own value systems and experience. Many parents share similar values and agree on which care is in the best interest of their child. For a variety of reasons, there may be conflict among family members about what is right for the child.

Physicians and other members of the health care team caring for these young children must assess the developmental level of each patient. The medical team should involve young patients in decisions whenever they are capable. This is particularly the case with pain management. The child should have the final say. Pain can be assessed using a rating scale appropriate for the age of the child to achieve a level of relief that is acceptable to the child (8).

Respect for an individual child also demands that we respond to their likes and dislikes as much as possible. Minimizing and relieving suffering and pain, as well as enhancing well being require knowledge of each patient as an individual. For example, is school important to the child and family and should every effort be expended to keep the child in school as long as possible? Or, does the patient have a history of school phobia and maximizing length of school attendance increases discomfort?

Children and adolescents with temporary guardians—Children may be with temporary guardians or in foster care as they approach the end of life. It is especially problematic when the courts, guardians, and foster parents are faced with end-of-life care decisions for a child who may die before the legal process rules whether the child will be returned to the custody of the parents. A do-not-resuscitate (DNR) order may be in the best interest of a patient. Physicians may need to approach the family court judge with legal responsibility for permission for medical care that is appropriate for the patient. For example, this would be the case for an infant whose head injuries are suspected to be from parental abuse. While the investigation is in progress, the patient may be a temporary ward of the state.

While medical decisions should always be in best interests of the child, it may be hard to identify who decides what these interests are in our pleuralistic society. Physicians must remember that they are responsible for making recommendations to a parent or guardian, and, except in emergency situations, lack the authority to decide medical care for a patient. Patients and their parents or guardians choose between medical options and what is important in life to them. When there is conflict, the hospital's Medical Ethics Committed may be consulted.

Palliative Care for Children

Pain control

The principles of pain management for children are similar to those for adult patients (Chapter 2). Pediatric patients and their families share many of the concerns about pain control that are prevalent in the adult medical community. There is concern about "addiction" to opioids needed to control pain and how to accurately assess pain. In addition, there are problems more specific to pediatrics. For example, long-acting opioid analgesics may not be available in dosages appropriate for young patients. School nurses and other personnel are reluctant to give pain medications in school. Immature, new teenage drivers frequently fail to appreciate why they should not continue driving while taking analgesics that can adversely affect motor and mental function. In dealing with patients and families in these situations, pediatricians cannot always facilitate resolutions that are safe, effective, and acceptable to all parties concerned. However, someone must take the responsibility to insure that someone on the team has addressed and reached consensus on the issues.

Nutrition and Fluids

The growing child who just maintains his weight and ceases to grow is regressing, not "holding his own." Nutrition, therefore, is of major importance for pediatricians, parents, children and adolescents, and their families. Many sub-specialty teams include nutritionists who help us maximize the patient's opportunities for growth. Supplemental formulas, nasogastric feedings, feeding buttons to facilitate enteral nutrition into the stomach, and total parenteral nutrition play a prominent role in pediatric care. Therefore, it is extremely difficult for many pediatricians to advise, or for patients and families to accept, that dying children often do not want to eat for a valid reason—they are not hungry. Allowing a child who is dying to control his own food and fluid intake can be a source of conflict in pediatric end-of-life care. The issues need to be addressed with sensitivity and concern for the patient's care and suffering.

Day care and school

The work of childhood is acquiring the informal and formal education that will enable each individual to maximize his potential. Young children benefit from contact with peers, teachers, and child care workers in a day care or preschool setting. Curricula in public or private schools or in the home school environment facilitate children's learning and development. School districts provide homebound teachers for students unable to attend school on a regular basis secondary to illness; pediatric inpatient facilities have certified teachers to work with young patients in these settings.

Many patients and families choose to participate in school re-entry programs coordinated and staffed by pediatric professionals that transition patients with potentially life-threatening illnesses back into the classroom during their therapy. School nurses, teachers and administrators, and support staff are generally unfamiliar with many of the chronic and life-threatening illnesses of childhood including cancer, renal disease, cystic fibrosis, and progressive neurological or neuromuscular diseases.

Other students are often unaware of what to expect and have a variety of concerns that lead to avoiding their sick classmate: They may be afraid the disease is "catching." They worry they might cause harm to a patient who looks cushingoid, pale, or has no hair. They are afraid that their friend will die.

Where palliative care is needed and death is approaching, counselors, teachers, and child life professionals involved in such programs often re-visit the classroom and/or staff to provide appropriate updates. Often there is need to answer questions and provide reassurance after the death of a child or adolescent for staff and students.

Extracurricular activities

Pediatric patients continue to participate in music and dance lessons, sports, or religious youth groups. They attend summer camps, belong to scouts or other clubs, or have jobs. Patients and families benefit from guidance from pediatricians and other members of the team as the clinical course evolves. Young children and adolescents may need encouragement to continue to participate as fully as possible. Medical issues must be addressed. For example, acute thrombocytopenia would prohibit a number of physical activities.

"Make-a-Wish"

Death in childhood or adolescence is not the norm. The patients, their families, and society as a whole recognize the tragedy of a foreshortened life. Death before adulthood may bring an end to suffering. But it never comes at the end of a long, full life.

There are many organizations, including the Make-a-Wish Foundation, which offer children with potentially life-threatening illnesses the opportunity to have a dream fulfilled. The child may wish for and receive a computer that allows him to acquire new skills, gives him a new window on the world, and affords him opportunities to interact with his siblings. The child may be granted a trip with her family to visit grandparents she has never met or go to a theme park for a week of fun. These opportunities to broaden their horizons are extremely important to many children, their families, and those who work toward being able to grant wishes for them. Physicians caring for these patients must certify that they meet medical criteria and that the activity is safe and appropriate.

Goals of End-of-Life Care in Pediatrics

The goals of end-of-life care in pediatrics are in accord with those espoused by the World Health Organization. Pediatricians continue to affirm life, regard dying as a normal process, neither hasten nor postpone death, provide relief from pain and other symptoms, and integrate psychological and spiritual care through use of an interdisciplinary team (9). However, pediatricians must also acknowledge that death during infancy, childhood, and adolescence is associated with its own set of issues for patients, parents, and those caring for them. It is the careful attention to the uniqueness of the maturing patient that can facilitate the best possible relief of suffering during the dying process.

References

1. National Center for Health Statistics Public Use File, 1997.
2. Leikin S. A proposal concerning decisions to forego life-sustaining treatment for young people. J Pediatr 1989;115:17–22.
3. Appelbaum PS, Grisso T. Assessing patients' capacities to consent to treatment. N Engl J Med 1988;319:1635–1638.
4. Holder AR. Disclosure and consent; problems in pediatrics. Law, Medicine and Health Care 1988;16:3–4 and 219–228.
5. Sigman GS, O'Connor C. Exploration for physicians of the mature minor doctrine. J Pediatr 1991;119:520–525.
6. Freyer DR. Children with cancer: special considerations in the discontinuation of life-sustaining treatment. Med Pediatr Oncol 1992;20:136–142.
7. Children Oncology Group Bioethics Committee recommendation, 2001.
8. Wong DL. Whaley and Wong's essentials of pediatric nursing. 5th ed. St. Louis: Mosby, 1995.
9. World Health Organization, 1990 (from the AMA EPEC course materials: Elements and models of end-of-life care, Definition 2, 1999).

Additional reading:

Berde CB, Sethna NF. Analgesics for the treatment of pain in children. N Engl J Med 2002;347:1094–1103.

11

Dying of Old Age: The Frail Nursing Home Resident

George J. Taylor and Jerome E. Kurent

There are more people living today aged 65 years and older than in the history of our planet. People in the developed world are living healthier and older than ever before. The average American died at age 46 at the turn of the twentieth century. In the US, men now live an average 75 years, and women, 77 years. One-half of the women alive today will live until 85 years of age, and the number of centenarians has doubled from 1980 to 1990.

A century ago, 90% of deaths occurred as a consequence of acute illness or trauma. Today, 90% of deaths are the result of chronic illness (see Chapter 1). A related development is that most people now have the opportunity to express their preferences for care during late life and terminal illness. Advance directives facilitate this option and are a modern innovation.

The term, elderly, arbitrarily refers to individuals 65 years of age and older. People 85 years and older are defined as the *very old*, and represent the fastest growing segment of the US population. They experience at least a 20% incidence of dementia (Chapter 6), and most eventually require nursing home care. Approximately half of the US population will spend at least some time in a long-term care facility. Twenty-five percent of deaths in this country now occur in long-term care facilities, and this is expected to increase with our aging population.

Can we expect adequate end-of-life care as a standard of care in the long-term care setting in the foreseeable future? Changes in public policy will be needed if there is to be funding for adequate palliative and end-of-life care for the aging baby boomers and subsequent generations. The benefits of long-term health insurance in meeting these needs are presently limited to individuals with adequate finances to fund this option.

How nursing homes work and are regulated

The families of elderly patients who recently died report more dissatisfaction with the nursing home than any other environment where death takes place (1). Despite its obvious role as the final stop for many who have chronic life-limiting illness, American nursing homes have focused on "rehabilitative" rather than palliative care (2).

This emphasis on rehabilitation had its origin in the early 1980s when studies documented poor quality of care in nursing homes. These revelations prompted the US Congress to pass reform legislation which included specific goals and standards of care (3). At that time in American medicine, there was seemingly little appreciation for the value of palliative care, and the focus of new regulations was on restoring function whenever possible. Since then, federal and state regulations have graded nursing homes on their potential to rehabilitate residents.

Such regulations may serve to impede the provision of high quality of care at the end of life. As an example, federal guidelines for many of the signs and symptoms of terminal illness identify them as treatable. Weight loss, progressive loss of function, and the development of bowel and bladder incontinence can be inevitable consequences of end-stage medical illness. Failure to implement care plans to correct these problems—even in the dying patient—may be cited by external reviewers as deficiencies of the nursing home, even though such efforts are usually inappropriate for a dying patient (4).

Death occurring in the nursing home has frequently been used as a negative statistic by external reviewers. This denies the fact that the majority of nursing home residents are actually expected to die from the complex and disabling conditions requiring their admission. Active rehabilitation efforts are rewarded with the highest per diem payment, while palliative care receives lower reimbursement. There is an obvious need to modify long-term care policies and regulations to more accurately reflect the needs of nursing home patients, many of whom are at the end of life.

Nursing homes operate on limited budgets, and yet are expected to comply with increasingly strict regulatory and reimbursement guidelines. It is therefore not surprising that these facilities have been slow to implement new programs focusing on palliative care. Like anything new, they may be perceived as cumbersome and adding to the cost burden, although in reality palliative care and hospice care are usually cost effective (4,5).

Pain management and the nursing home resident: under-treatment and non-treatment of pain

The nursing home resident often has a few strikes against her (the female:male ratio is 4:1), with clinical features that may be obstacles to implementation of palliative care. She is more likely to die of a non-cancer diagnosis. The 6-month prognosis guidelines for hospice eligibility for patients with non-cancer diagnoses are sometimes more challenging to predict than for patients with cancer (6). Physicians are much more likely to enroll cancer patients in hospice than those with non-cancer diagnoses, although this is gradually changing.

The nursing home resident frequently has some cognitive impairment. This may be associated with suboptimal assessment of pain, and result in undertreatment or non-treatment of pain. When the patient is confused, doctors either fail to recognize pain or are reluctant to use pain-relieving drugs.

Studies have indicated that 25% to 40% of nursing home residents have untreated or undertreated pain. Patients at greatest risk for undertreatment of pain include those who are older than 85 years, of male gender, have cognitive impairment, or are ethnic minorities (7). Assessment of pain in the geriatric patient is often inadequate or not done at all.

Frail geriatric patients may not be able to express the fact that they are in pain. Patients with dementia may express pain by non-verbal means, including grimacing, fidgeting, frowning, groaning, or heavy breathing. Agitation which may be attributed to underlying dementia may actually be a primary manifestation of pain.

More recently, "pain as a 5th vital sign" is being adopted by medical institutions as a standard to reinforce the need to assess all patients for pain. Pain assessment instruments, such as the Likert scale 0–10 are used effectively in adult, cognitively intact patients. Zero indicates no pain, while 10 indicates the worst pain imaginable. Cognitively impaired patients may not be able to use this instrument. Choosing from a succession of faces, from smiling to frowning, may be more appropriate for assessing the impaired patient.

The elderly patient's expectations may influence pain management. If there is belief that old age naturally means suffering and pain, there may be reluctance for the geriatric patient to request pain medication. Box 11-1 describes an interview that illustrates this point. An elderly person's reduced expectations for pain control may be based on years of observing friends and family members die painful deaths. Some may have firm religious beliefs suggesting that "this suffering may be God's will." Sadly, many patients have also been told by their physicians during times of less severe illness that pain is an inevitable part of

BOX 11-1

An interview with the surviving wife of a patient who died a painful death due to metastatic colon carcinoma, illustrating reduced expectations for pain control in the elderly

Mrs S. is an intelligent, engaging woman in her late 70s whose husband died at age 80 from metastatic colon carcinoma after 2 years of unsuccessful treatment. She agreed to a clinical study which included an extensive "after-death interview instrument for family-member survivors" 12 months after her husband's death. She was asked about pain control during the last two weeks of life.

Interviewer: "Did your husband experience any pain during the last 2 weeks of life, and for what percentage of time?"

Deceased patient's wife: "Oh, he had pain and for much more than 50% of the time. I mean he had pain all the time. The last 3 days the pain never stopped . . ."

Interviewer: (later during the interview) "On a scale of 1 to 10, how would you rate your husband's care during the last weeks and days of his life?"

Answer, "I would rate it a '10'—it was excellent! Everybody did everything they could."

Interviewer: "But I understood that he had unrelieved pain during most of his dying days."

Answer, "He did, but this is what you expect when you get old and then die. This is what our friends have experienced, and that's just how it is."

Interviewer: "But you understood that there are powerful medications to treat pain—why shouldn't they be used?"

Answer, "Well my husband and I are religious people, and this dying pain could be God's will. My husband just did not want to interfere and did not ask for more medicine."

the aging process, reducing expectations for pain control during terminal illness.

Not surprisingly, younger members of the same families are equally adamant that pain relief must be provided for themselves if pain were to occur. These inter-generational differences in expectations for pain control are often dramatic.

A challenge to primary care clinicians is to educate all of our patients that there are effective means to control pain, and to advocate for the appropriate use of potent analgesic medications. Remember, between 90% to 95% of pain can be adequately managed, regardless of the etiology and the patient's age.

Treatment of acute illness

The nursing home resident's proximate cause of death could be a potentially treatable condition, such as aspiration pneumonia or urinary tract infection. Physicians often feel compelled to treat conditions that are easily cured, even in patients with underlying severe life-limiting or terminal conditions.

All too frequently, when the nursing home resident with severe life-limiting disease develops fever, she is transferred to the acute care hospital, initially in the emergency department by physicians who do not know her family. Advance directives are often non-existent, and there may not be a do-not-resuscitate (DNR) order. This sets the stage for treatment that does little more than prolong the dying process. It is an unfortunate chain of events that could be prevented with careful attention to end of life planning. This is usually initiated by the primary care doctor (Chapter 1), and it should be a part of the doctor's checklist whenever admitting a patient to a nursing home.

Hospice and the nursing home

A 1999 study determined that 70% of nursing homes had no patients enrolled in a hospice program, despite the fact that hospice programs maximize care for terminally-ill patients and their families (2).

Because of changing expectations more nursing home patients are choosing hospice services. Medicare now allows reimbursement for hospice care, even though the patient is on a nursing unit (8). There are a number of significant advantages that are associated with hospice care (Chapter 1).

The hospice patient has a better chance of getting adequate palliation. The hospice nurse oversees therapy, insuring that medicines are given at effective doses and using the proper route of administration (i.e., subcutaneous rather than intramuscular injection when parenteral therapy is needed). Useless therapies are avoided, including feeding tubes and antibiotics. The rate of unwanted hospitalization decreases (and with this, the cost of care) (4,5,9).

An important practical advantage of hospice care is its psychological impact on all caregivers. With hospice involved, everyone understands that life-prolonging treatment will be avoided, and caregivers are thus comfortable with the palliative model of care. Without hospice enrollment, the patient has a less well-defined status and is more likely to receive aggressive care, even when advance directives proscribe it. Hospice status thus protects the patient, ensuring that a desire for comfort care will be honored.

Hospice also helps the family. It's stated "care unit" includes the patient and the family caregiver. In contrast, the nursing home, like the hospital, tends to consider the family "visitors." (Perhaps this is an overstatement, but you know what we are getting at.) Few nursing homes provide bereavement services, a standard component of hospice care.

Failure to thrive—a nursing home diagnosis

Those of us who practice in acute care hospitals are used to helping terminally-ill patients with an obviously diseased organ system: heart, lung, or kidney disease or cancer of something. There are also elderly patients in nursing homes who slowly dwindle and die. "Failure to thrive" is a term that describes patients experiencing weight loss and decline leading to death.

There may be a combination of illnesses that ultimately lead to death. Some have an element of dementia or another neurologic illness (see Chapter 6). Osteoarthritis and compression fractures, common in elderly women, may cause pain. Reduced oral intake, weight loss, and progressive loss of function lead to death. Without tube feeding and hydration, the patient dies peacefully.

Can aggressive pain relief and withholding tube feeding be interpreted as euthanasia? We think not. The moral imperative is to provide relief of suffering. A family witnessing the terrible pain of a loved one quickly appreciates the need for palliation. When pain is not adequately treated, the family may be left with guilt, and with negative feelings toward a health care system that could have, but did not, relieve suffering.

Walk into any nursing home today, and you will find residents who are incurably ill being tube fed, unable to communicate, usually incontinent, and requiring total care. The family may visit frequently at first, but the frequency diminishes when it is clear that the elderly patient is no longer aware of his/her surroundings.

| BOX 11-2 | *A conversation with the family of an 82-year-old woman who has stopped eating** |

"It is important that we are meeting today, because we have important decisions to make for your mother. She has entrusted you with the responsibility to make these decisions, and you 'speak with her voice.'

"She has stopped eating and drinking. Her back pain was terrible. We finally got the dose of the pain medicine where it is working, and she is now sleeping most of the time. Based on what has happened over the last few months, I do not think the pain will improve with time, and believe we will need to continue the medicine.

"Here is the new problem: with this level of pain control she no longer wants food. She is taking in a little, but it is not enough for her to live on. The decision, now, is whether we should feed her artificially. This would require putting a feeding tube into her stomach, either through her nose, or surgically through the wall of her stomach. Twenty years ago I might have urged you to do this, but I do not feel that way now.

"The medical ethics experts talk of it this way: when a creature in nature loses its ability to eat and drink, that fact defines the end of life. We are all creatures of nature, and when we no longer wish to eat, that also defines the end of our natural lives. We now feel that it is of doubtful value for the doctors and nurses to feed a person artificially, especially when that person cannot get well. In that case, all we are doing is making the dying process longer and more uncomfortable. We are not helping the person to get well.

"The next question is whether your mother will suffer because she is eating and drinking little. There is a lot of experience with this, as this is a common way that elderly people die. What happens is that the person sleeps a lot, waking on occasion. They rarely ask for food or water—and of course, if they do, we provide it. They just do not seem hungry or thirsty, and there seems to be very little suffering. They die peacefully.

"It would seem this would happen quickly for a person as old and frail as your mother, and we cannot accurately predict the timing of death. But in some cases it can go on as long as a couple weeks. What I can promise to do for her and for you is to provide good comfort care. If you feel she is having pain that is not controlled, we will adjust the medicine to make it better. I will stay with her and with you through this."

---

* This may be modified to apply in any case where oral intake has stopped.

The "patient" is then "maintained" by technicians who are strangers. This is not what we would desire for ourselves as our lives wind down. Rather, it seems an undignified and cruel distortion of our humanity, courtesy of modern medicine.

Be aware that starting a tube feeding is not an irreversible decision. Like other life-support interventions (i.e., mechanical ventilation or dialysis), it can be considered a therapeutic trial. If the patient fails to improve it may be stopped. There is no moral or ethical distinction between withdrawing and withholding such interventions.

Box 11-2 records a conversation with a patient's family that reviews present attitudes about tube feeding and hydration, and it applies to any patient with terminal illness who has stopped eating or drinking. It also reflects our desire to allow those who may be "dying from old age" to do so peacefully.

The experience of terminal illness: what really matters

There is a growing appreciation of the role of spirituality in helping to achieve a good death (10). Taking a "spiritual history" may help. The FICA spiritual assessment has been suggested. The acronym FICA includes F (Faith, Belief, Meaning); I (Importance and Influence); C (Community); and A (Address/Action in Care), and can be of great value when used with your patients nearing the end of life.

Geriatric patients often indicate a need to achieve spiritual peace as they near the end of life. This process can be difficult if the physician is preoccupied with a cure. Conflict and distress are inevitable when the physician refuses to accept that a cure is no longer possible, especially when the family buys into unrealistic hopes. Persisting with futile interventions may distract the patient and family from important end-of-life work.

Achieving spiritual peace presupposes resolving problems in the family or with friends. This requires communication involving all stakeholders. The sensitive clinician often is the one who initiates the process of open discussion that involves the patient, family, friends, clergy, and caregivers.

References

1. Zerzan J, Stearns S, Hanson L. Access to palliative care and hospice in nursing homes. JAMA 2000;284:2489–2494.
2. Hanson L, Danis M, Garrett J. What is wrong with end-of-life care? Opinions of bereaved family members. J Am Geriatr Soc 1997;45: 1339–1344.

3. Phillips C, Morris J, Hawes C, et al. Association of the Resident Assessment Instrument (RAI) with changes in function, cognition and psychosocial status. J Am Geriatr Soc 1997;45:986–993.

4. Petrisek A, Mor V. Hospice in nursing homes: a facility-level analysis of the distribution of hospice beneficiaries. Gerontologist 1999;39: 279–290.

5. Baer W, Hanson L. Families' perceptions of the added value of hospice in the nursing home. J Am Geriatr Soc 2000;48:879–882.

6. Fox E, Landrum-McNiff K, Xhong Z, et al. Evaluations of prognostic criteria for determining hospice eligibility in patients with advanced lung, heart or liver disease (SUPPORT). JAMA 1999;282:1638–1645.

7. Won A, Lapane K, Gambassi G, et al. Correlates and management of non-malignant pain in the nursing home. J Am Geriatr Soc 1999;47: 936–942.

8. Christakis N, Escarce J. Survival of Medicare patients after enrollment in hospice programs. N Engl J Med 1996;335:172–178.

9. Watt C. Hospices within nursing homes: should a long-term care facility wear both hats? Am J Hosp Palliat Care 1997;14:63–65.

10. Puchalski CM, Romer AL. Taking a spiritual history allows clinicians to understand patients more fully. J Pall Med 2000;3:129–137.

Index